Vitality & Vitals

This Journal Belongs To:

Name:

Home Phone:

Cell:

Work Phone:

Address:

Email:

In case of emergency call:

Family Doctor:

Pharmacy:

Provincial Health Care Number:

Other Health Insurance:

I have the following medical alert conditions:

I am allergic to:

www.vitalityandvitals.com

Please visit our website to give us your feedback and comments. You will also find locations where the journal is available.

Learn the basics of a balanced lifestyle.

Keep track of your health history, health concerns, appointments and treatments.

Here's to your best health!

Canadian Version

For adults 18 and up

Vitality & Vitals
My health and lifestyle journal

Beverly Whitmore
Lorna Milkovich

The opinions expressed in this journal are those of the authors. You are advised to consult a medical doctor before acting on the basis of material contained in this journal. The authors hereby disclaim any responsibility for any loss suffered by a person, which results from a failure to consult a medical doctor.

Calgary 2005

Published by Vitality & Vitals Inc.

Manufactured in Canada

Cover and book design by Vangool Design & Typography

Library and Archives Canada Cataloguing in Publication

Whitmore, Beverly, 1952-

Vitality & vitals / Beverly Whitmore, Lorna Milkovich.

ISBN 0-9737766-0-9

1. Medical records. 2. Health. 3. Diaries (Blank-books)

I. Milkovich, Lorna, 1958- II. Title. III. Title: Vitality and vitals.

R864.W49 2005 613 C2005-901671-X

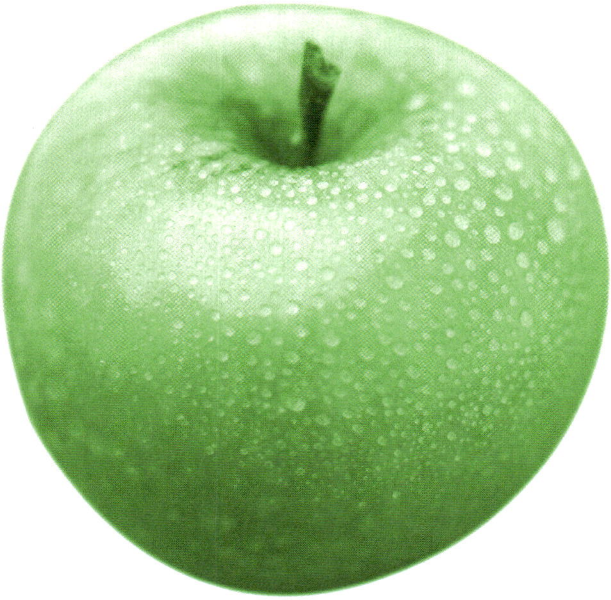

"Knowing is not enough, we must apply. Willing is not enough, we must do."

GOETHE, POET, PLAYWRIGHT, NOVELIST

What is in this journal for you?

Are you enjoying life to the fullest? Do you have energy and stamina to meet life's challenges? Or are habits such as eating too much, doing too much, sleeping too little, and having too little fun draining your physical and mental energy; your vitality? Did you know that these habits also have an enormous effect on your long-term health?

"Health is a state of physical, mental and social wellbeing, not merely an absence of diseases or infirmity."

World Health Organization

Vitality & Vitals is a unique combination of a vitality journal and a health journal.

In the **Vitality** section you will assess your daily habits and learn how simple improvements can add energy to your days and better health to your years.

In the **Vitals** section you will keep track of your health history, health concerns, appointments and treatments. You won't be stuck trying to recall details of your health months or years later. Your health details will be at your fingertips.

Track your health over time to assess general trends. If you're responsible for keeping track of your children's, spouse's, or parents' health appointments and health history you will want a Vitality & Vitals journal for each of them.

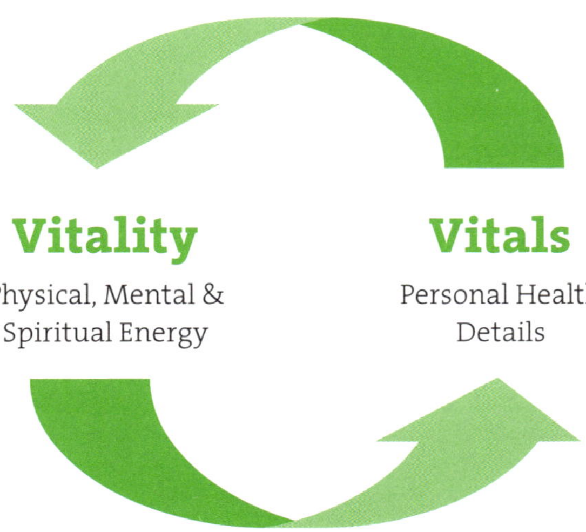

Our motivation for writing this journal

As health professionals, we've noticed that people often can't remember details of their health history such as medications or dates of surgeries. We asked friends, colleagues and family how they kept track of their health details, but most of their systems were haphazard. The best system we found was the scribblers our mothers use to jot down important details. This helped to plant the seed to design an organized and comprehensive journal — VITALS.

It was only natural to include VITALITY in the journal. Most of our careers have been about counselling people with high blood pressure, high cholesterol and other conditions to live healthier lives. We've written a best selling workbook on the subject: Taking Control of Your Blood Pressure: Steps to a Healthier Lifestyle. We know that healthy life-styles not only lower our chances of developing many diseases, but also improve the quality of our lives.

We often lose sight of the importance of health until illness strikes. Yet many of us are functioning far below our maximum potential, not realizing we can feel a whole lot better. We strongly believe in the personal power each and every one of us has to feel our very best.

We are passionate about the combined Vitality & Vitals journal because of its potential to help improve the vitality and long-term health of each person using it! To your best health!

Beverly Whitmore, BSc, RD, MBA

Lorna Milkovich, RN, BN, MBA

"Instead of looking at life as a narrowing funnel, we can see it ever widening to choose the things we want to do, to take the wisdom we've learned and create something."

LIZ CARPENTER, WRITER

We would like to thank our family, friends and colleagues who kindly offered us their support and feedback.

Icon Key

- General Information
- Important/Caution
- Actions to Take

Contents

"It is not enough to be busy. The question is: what are you busy about?"

HENRY DAVID THOREAU, AUTHOR, POET & PHILOSOPHER

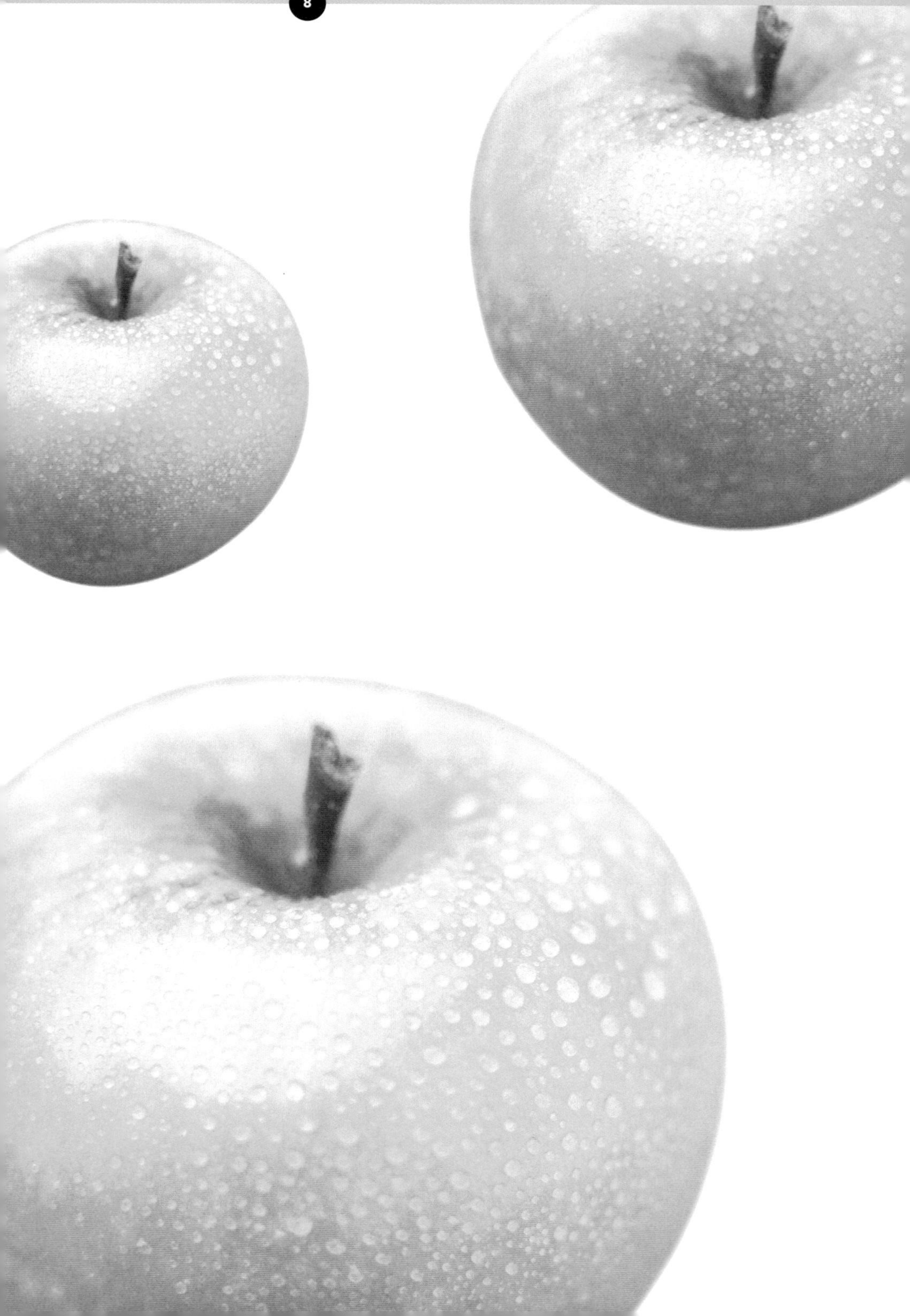

Vitality

"Right now you are one choice away from a new beginning — one that leads you toward becoming the fullest human being you can be."

OPRAH WINFREY

What is Vitality?

Vitality is a balance between your physical, mental and spiritual energy. Everyday choices you make, from the food you eat to the amount you sleep, affect your vitality. These lifestyle choices also affect your health and longevity.

In the Vitality section of this journal you'll learn ways to:

- **Balance Your Life**
  It all starts with balance between your body, mind and spirit.
- **Recharge Your Eating Habits**
  Compare your diet with the healthy eating guidelines and map out a healthy intake for you.
- **Revitalize Your Days with Activity**
  Work activity into your days.
- **Refresh Your Life with Sleep**
  Learn how to improve your sleep, one of the most undervalued, yet key ingredients to vitality.
- **Be a Healthy Weight**
  Throw out the fad diets and get down to the basics of achieving a healthy weight.
- **Rethink Alcohol, Tobacco, and Drugs**
  Live free from the control of substances.
- **Rate Your Vitality**
  Use a simple 5-point scale to rate your lifestyle.

Heredity accounts for only 25 percent of how long people live. The other 75 percent is due to lifestyle.

Dr. Walter Willett, Eat Drink and Be Healthy 2001

Balance Your Life

Need to balance your life?

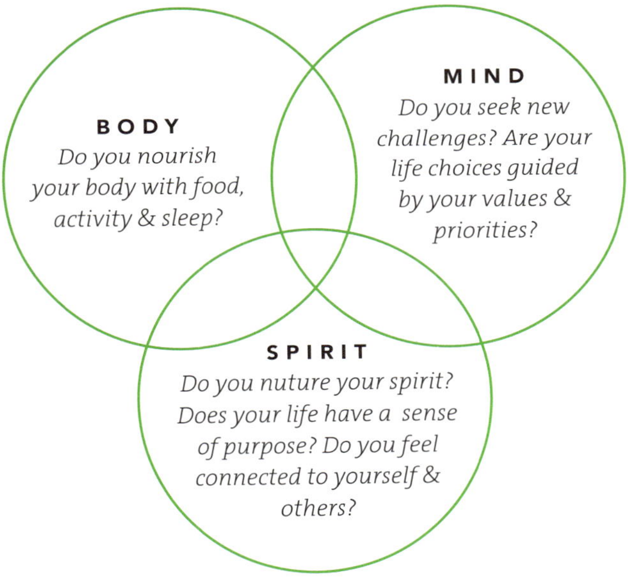
BODY
Do you nourish your body with food, activity & sleep?
MIND
Do you seek new challenges? Are your life choices guided by your values & priorities?
SPIRIT
Do you nuture your spirit? Does your life have a sense of purpose? Do you feel connected to yourself & others?

Changing life circumstances such as marriage, divorce, birth of a child and job loss constantly push us to find a new 'balance' in our lives. What aspects of your vitality are the strongest? What aspects are you neglecting?

Reality Bites

too much work

25 percent of Canadians work more than 50 hours a week, compared with 10 percent a decade ago.

too little time

Our lives tend to be thrown out of balance by doing too many things in too little time and letting the

"Your vision will become clear only when you look into your heart. Who looks outside, dreams. Who looks inside, awakens."

CARL JUNG,
PSYCHIATRIST

"Laughter is the brush that sweeps away the cobwebs of the heart."

MORT WALKER,
CARTOONIST

"Joy is not in things - it's in us."

RICHARD WAGNER, COMPOSER AND AUTHOR

Symptoms of Depression:

Poor concentration or difficulty making decisions

Poor appetite or overeating

Sleeping too much or too little

Low energy or tiredness

Low self esteem

Feelings of helplessness

expectations of others pressure us. Time stress was the biggest concern of Canadians in 2004.

too much tv

The number one leisure activity of Canadians is watching television. The average weekly time spent watching television is 22 hours, according to a Statistics Canada survey.

too much stress

Certain situations can provoke stress, but our thoughts determine whether or not they are a problem for us. The same situation can motivate one person and stress another person.

Too much stress or poorly handled stress can lead to tiredness, anxiety, memory loss, increased susceptibility to colds and flu, difficulty sleeping, errors in judgment and personality changes. Eventually, stress can lead to long-term illness.

too much depression

An estimated 25 percent of Canadians have a degree of depression serious enough to need treatment at some time in their lives.

too little knowledge

A 2001 Compas survey found 91 percent of Canadians say maintaining their mental health is very important. But one in four doesn't know how to maintain and improve his/her mental health.

Keys to finding balance in your life

choose simplicity

Simplify your life based on your priorities and values. You will find that it is possible to need less, want less, spend less and feel more at peace.

live by your values

What are the things you value most? Often money and career take precedence, leaving the rest of our lives out of balance. Yet it is often the other aspects of our lives that give us the most personal satisfaction.

priorize

Notice how you spend your time and money in order to discover what your real priorities are. Are you happy with these choices, or is it time to rethink your priorities?

people in your life

Surround yourself with people who energize you and help you to feel good about yourself.

cherish your time

Create more time in your life for things that matter to you and let go of the rest.

live in the moment

Enjoy the moment rather than focusing on the future or the past. The past is gone; the future is yet to be.

foster inner growth

Cultivate inner growth and spirituality through practices such as meditation, prayer, yoga, reading, journal writing and time for inner reflection.

Simplify Your Life

Do only the things you love or need to do

Unclutter your house, keep only what you love or need

Don't over schedule and over commit

Surround yourself with people who give energy rather than drain it

Always live guided by your values and integrity

When choosing to do something, first ask yourself:

Why am I doing this?

What will I accomplish?

Will this make me happy?

Treat yourself to something you love to do at least once every week.

"Let us make one point, that we meet each other with a smile, when it is difficult to smile. Smile at each other, make time for each other in your family."

MOTHER THERESA IN HER NOBEL PRIZE LECTURE

immerse yourself in nature

Notice the pure joy and calm you experience in nature. Take time to get back to nature: go for a walk, hike, ski or bike ride. Bring nature inside by creating spaces reflective of nature.

adopt a pet

Pets provide countless hours of joy, entertainment and unconditional love. Most people don't understand the value of pets and their companionship until they get one. But only get a pet if you are ready, willing and able to provide it with a good quality of life. They need play, exercise and outdoor time, along with the basic necessities.

laugh

If you haven't laughed for a while you may have forgotten how good it makes you feel. Loosen up by seeing a comedy show or reading the comics in the newspaper. Laughing at yourself takes some of the pressure out of difficult situations.

"The instant Pierre, the little feline ball of fur, decided to settle in my lap for a nap, purring all the while, I could literally feel the tension leave my body, and I was overwhelmed by a feeling of utter serenity."

AMBA BALU, FAMILY PHYSICIAN

The road ahead

simplify and create balance in your life

By being conscious of the need to find balance in your life it will become more natural to live by your values and priorities.

Use your personal power to make choices based upon your priorities and values.

Ask yourself:

- **What are my values?** For example, health, family, security, peace of mind and spirituality.
- **What are my priorities?** Notice if they are in sync with what you value.
- **What would it take to make my priorities match my values?**
- **How would I like my life to look?** For example, family, friends, job, and adventure.
- **What can I eliminate from my life?**
- **What do I need to add to my life?**
- **What would I do if I weren't afraid of failing?**
- **What is one thing I can do every week to treat myself?**

My daily walks are a peaceful time to energize myself. Every problem I encounter seems smaller and the solution comes easier during a good walk.

Beverly

"Do... or do not. There is no try."

YODA, STAR WARS

My answers:

Recharge Your Eating Habits

Need to recharge your eating habits?

Are your eating habits energizing your life and setting you up for good long-term health? Our eating habits are often the first to suffer when we get too busy or stressed, especially if they weren't that healthy in the first place. Mealtime should be respected as a time to break from other activities, fuel our bodies and enjoy the company of others.

The ultimate food intake:

- provides energy
- is pleasing and satisfying
- meets the body's energy and nutrient needs
- minimizes the risk of chronic disease

Dr. Walter Willett, Eat Drink and Be Healthy 2001

Reality Bites

Canadians are changing their eating habits

A Tracking Nutrition Trends survey found almost 65 percent of Canadians changed their diet for the better in 2003. They wanted to feel better, to lose weight and to stay healthy for old age.

food protects

Healthy eating provides energy and nutrients and lowers your risk of developing chronic diseases such as heart disease, diabetes and osteoporosis.

breakfast skippers miss out

People who skip breakfast take in less calcium, iron, fibre and energy. These key nutrients are found in breakfast foods. Intake of these nutrients is usually not made up at other meals.

"Our truest life is when we are in our dreams awake!"

HENRY DAVID THOREAU, AUTHOR, POET & PHILOSOPHER

a perfect food doesn't exist

More than 50 nutrients are needed for growth, repair and maintenance of the body. No one food or food group provides all of these nutrients. Canada's Food Guide recommends a variety from four food groups to help you to get the nutrients that you require.

grocery stores can be overwhelming

There are more than 50,000 items in a large grocery store. It is easy to get sidetracked without a shopping list.

portion sizes on food labels can be tricky

The Nutrition Facts on food labels present accurate information in a standard form that allows consumers to compare products. However, serving sizes listed may be smaller than what you would consume. For example, a popular brand of frozen pizza lists a serving as being one-sixth of a nine-inch pizza.

Keys to recharging your eating habits

plan ahead

Most families rotate 10 different recipes. Think about what your 10 are and how they contribute to your vitality.

Try planning simple menus including the four food groups for a week at a time. Planning can help to avoid last minute unhealthy choices.

Make a grocery list from your menu.

The Four Food Groups:

- Grain Products
- Vegetables & Fruit
- Milk Products
- Meat & Alternatives

Portion Control

As a general rule avoid portions larger than your fist.

My 10 recipies:

divide your plate

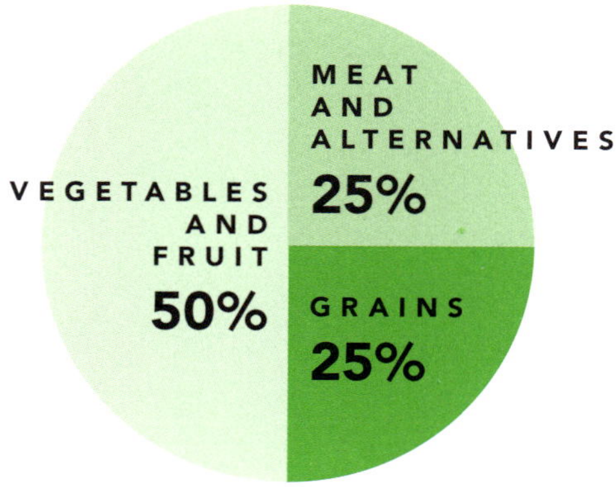

Here's a simple way to balance your meal: fill your plate with one quarter meat or alternative protein source, one quarter grain products and one half vegetables and fruit.

eat for a healthy weight

It's no surprise that super sized servings will make you super sized. Downsize your servings by:

- **Ordering half portions or senior meals in restaurants.**
- **Deciding how much of the food on your plate you will eat** and pushing the rest to the side before you start.
- **Avoiding the use of oversized dishes at home.** Don't use a plate over 10" in diameter. You should be able to see a one inch rim around the plate.

choose whole grains

Whole and less refined grains are more nutritious and contain more fibre than refined grains. The body takes longer to digest whole grains, keeping blood sugar levels lower. This helps to decrease hunger,

Whole Grain Choices:

- whole grain breads
- whole grain cereals
- barley
- bulgur
- brown rice
- old fashioned oatmeal
- popcorn

Look for whole grain or 100 percent whole before the name of the grain on the food label.

making weight control easier.

Regular use of whole grains is linked to a lower risk of heart disease, diabetes and some cancers.

Make a point of eating whole grains three or more times each day.

choose fibre

Most people only consume about half of the fibre recommended. To increase your fibre intake, read labels and choose high fibre products.

We all know that fibre is good for us, but did you know that there are two kinds of fibre: soluble and insoluble?

- **Soluble fibre** is found in foods such as oats, barley, psyllium, fruits and vegetables, beans and lentils. It lowers cholesterol, controls appetite, and evens out blood sugar levels. These foods also contain some insoluble fibre.
- **Insoluble fibre** found in foods such as bran and whole wheat helps to keep your bowels regular. These foods also contain some soluble fibre.

go for color

The vividly coloured fruits and vegetables contain essential vitamins, minerals, fibre and phytochemicals that your body needs for health. The more colour, the more health benefits you get.

Fresh, canned, dried or frozen fruits and vegetables all add valuable nutrients to your diet. Make fruits and vegetables part of every meal and your number one snack choice.

Goal Fibre Intakes

ADULT WOMEN
21-25 grams per day

ADULT MEN
30-38 grams per day

Examples of Fibre in Foods

FOOD	FIBRE CONTENT (GRAMS)
Whole grain bread slice	2 g
High fibre cereals	5 g or more
Medium apple or pear	4 g
1/2 cup navy beans, lentils or chickpeas	5 to 8 g

Constipation becomes more of a problem with age, affecting 25 percent of older men and 33 percent of older women.

Your Calcium Needs

Age 19 to 50
about 1,000 mg

Over 50 years
about 1,200 mg

FOOD	CALCIUM (MILLIGRAMS)
50 grams (1 3/4 oz) firm cheese	350
1 cup milk	350
3/4 cup fruit flavoured yoghurt	300
1/2 cup almonds	240
1/2 tin (213 g) salmon	200
1/2 cup broccoli	35
8 small sardines	165

Food is the best source of calcium.

Caution: Do not take more than 2,500 mg of calcium per day from food and supplements combined.

Sources of Omega-3 fatty acids:

- Fish: salmon, herring, sardines and albacore tuna
- Vegetable: soybean oil, flaxseeds, flaxseed oil, walnuts and canola oil

get your calcium

Calcium is necessary for healthy bones. Drink milk or eat milk-based products or other calcium-enriched sources such as soy or supplements daily.

You need more calcium and vitamin D after age 50. Calculate your calcium intake using the side bar, or even better, obtain a detailed calcium calculator chart from your doctor, pharmacist or dietitian. If your intake is under the recommendations consider first increasing food sources and secondly discuss the use of a supplement with your doctor or dietitian.

choose healthy protein foods

Protein is needed for tissue growth, maintenance and repair. Eat beans or lentils, fish, nuts, eggs and moderate portions of lean meats. Limit the use of high fat meats.

use healthy fats

Healthy fats provide energy, essential fatty acids and fat-soluble vitamins. Include sources of omega-3 fatty acids from fish and plant sources. Fats also add flavour to foods and help you to feel full.

seek great flavour

Flavour tends to satisfy your appetite with less food. Use ripened fruits and vegetables, and allow herbs and spices time to simmer for great flavour. Limit your use of salt.

While travelling in Thailand I noticed that very few Thais are overweight. The intense flavour of their food satisfies their appetite with smaller quantities. Lorna

choose water first

Water is the original thirst quencher and should be your number one drink choice. Water is needed to digest food, for healthy skin, and to keep every system in your body healthy. We look better and have more energy when we are well hydrated. Lack of water can lead to dehydration. Even mild dehydration can zap your energy.

tune into your water needs

Drink a glass of water with each meal and between each meal. Drink more water when you are active, in hot weather, and if you are pregnant or breast-feeding. You also likely need more water if you have the flu.

There isn't a daily-recommended water intake that fits for everyone. But you are probably drinking enough water if you quench your thirst, produce urine that is slightly yellow or colourless and feel well. However, as you age you are less able to sense when you are thirsty.

see your doctor

Check with your doctor or a registered dietitian if you're concerned about drinking too much or too little water. Increased thirst and increased urination can be signs of diabetes. Your doctor may advise you to drink less water if you have a condition such as heart failure.

vary your food

Eating a variety of foods is the best way to get the essential nutrients. Don't get stuck in a rut of eating the same foods every day. Try a new fruit or vegetable, a new recipe, or an ethnic restaurant. Combine foods in new and interesting ways.

Choose Healthy Fats:

- oils
- soft, non-hydrogenated margarines
- fish
- nuts & seeds

Avoid Trans or Hydrogenated Fats:

These fats raise your chance of having a heart attack. They are found in some: solid margarines, shortenings, cookies, crackers, fast foods, cake mixes, snack foods, waffles, microwave popcorn, cereal or energy bars.

Signs & Symptoms of Dehydration:

- excessive thirst
- fatigue
- headache
- dry mouth
- little or no urination
- muscle weakness
- dizziness
- light headedness

Mayo Clinic

"There is more hunger for love and appreciation in this world than for bread."

MOTHER THERESA

"It's choice — not chance that determines your destiny."

JEAN NIDETCH, FOUNDER, WEIGHT WATCHERS INTERNATIONAL

eat more carefully as you age

Generally, older people need less food and fewer calories because of muscle loss and a lower activity level. It becomes a challenge to take in all of the nutrients; therefore, as you age your food choices become more important than ever.

cook healthy for one

Honour your health, even when you're cooking for yourself. Include all four food groups in your menu plan. Cook a full meal at least three times per week. Make extra so you'll have healthy leftovers. Having a friend or family member for dinner may motivate you to prepare a healthy meal.

The road ahead

consider ways to make your diet healthier

MY GOAL	WHAT I NEED TO DO	TIME TO ACHIEVE	CHECK-UPS
EXAMPLE: Eat Breakfast daily	Buy breakfast food Plan breakfast the night before Set alarm 15 min early	One month	Write down what I eat for breakfast. Review my progress each Saturday

Revitalize Your Days with Activity

Need an activity tune-up?

If you're not doing regular activity, chances are you're not in shape. It might be time to rethink your activity routines.

Reality Bites

adult Canadians are inactive

According to surveys from the Canadian Fitness and Lifestyle Research Institute, the majority of Canadians face an increased risk of chronic disease and premature death due to physical inactivity. Two-thirds of Canadians aged 25 to 55 are not physically active enough for good health.

activity benefits the body & mind & spirit

Brain

Physically active older adults are less likely to have dementia (senility) and a decrease in their brainpower.

Heart

Inactive people who begin a regular program of exercise lower their risk of a heart attack by 35 to 55 percent. This includes activities such as gardening or walking.

"Inactivity is as harmful to your health as smoking."

HEALTH CANADA

A study found that TV watching increased a person's risk of becoming obese and developing diabetes. It estimated that walking at least 30 minutes a day and limiting TV watching to less than 10 hours per week could eliminate 30 percent of new cases of obesity & 43 percent of new cases of diabetes.

–2003, Journal of the American Medical Association (JAMA)

"If it weren't for the fact that the TV set and the refrigerator are so far apart, some of us wouldn't get any exercise at all."

JOEY ADAMS, COMEDIAN

"Lack of activity destroys the good condition of every human being, while movement and methodical physical exercise save it and preserve it."

PLATO, GREEK PHILOSOPHER

"We don't stop playing because we grow old. We grow old because we stop playing."

GEORGE BERNARD SHAW

Bones

Regular weight bearing activity, such as walking, can stop and sometimes reverse bone mineral loss. Exercise combined with a high calcium diet is especially effective.

Muscle Strength

Muscle is lost with aging. Between the ages of 25 and 50 people lose about 10 percent of their muscle. This may explain why your weight may not have changed, but more of it is hanging around your middle.

Between the ages of 50 and 80 people lose another 30 percent of their muscle. Ever notice the skinny arms and legs of older people?

Flexibility

Stretching activity becomes more important with age. Over the span of working life, adults lose eight to ten centimetres of lower back and hip flexibility. Staying flexible can help you to stay independent as you age. Flexibility is needed for daily activities such as climbing in and out of a car or bathtub.

Sleep & Mood

In a 10-week Harvard Medical School study, exercise was found to significantly improve sleep and reduce symptoms of depression.

Mind

A Canadian Fitness and Lifestyle Research Institute study found that four months of regular physical activity made people feel more relaxed, energized, and better able to handle stress.

Spirit

Time set aside for activity can also be time to allow your mind to connect with your inner thoughts and feelings.

Keys to activity

be active for an hour a day

We used to think you needed to go to the gym to exercise. We now realize that working activity into daily routines will contribute to good health. Housework and yard work count as activity!

You can measure your activity through steps or time. Make a goal of accumulating 10,000 steps per day by using a pedometer, or be purposely active for an hour a day. It's never too late to increase your activity.

balance your activity

Take part in **endurance** (aerobic) activities 4 to 7 days per week to:

- help your heart, lungs and circulatory system stay healthy
- give yourself more energy

Take part in **flexibility** activities 4 to 7 days per week to:

- keep your muscles relaxed and your joints mobile

Caution:

Check with your doctor before increasing exercise.

Minutes Count

If you are just starting to exercise or have some limitations to exercise, be active for 10 minutes at a time and add it up towards your daily total.

Endurance (aerobic) activities:
walking, running, yard work, cycling, skating, continuous swimming, tennis, dancing

Flexibility activities:
gardening, mopping the floor, yard work, vacuuming, stretching exercises, T'ai Chi, golf, bowling, yoga, curling, dance

Strength building activities:
climbing stairs, exercises like abdominal curls and push-ups, carrying objects, weight/strength-training routines

"I skate where the puck is going to be, not where it has been."

WAYNE GRETZKY

Take part in **strength** activities 2 to 4 days per week to:

- help your muscles and bones stay strong
- improve your posture
- help to prevent diseases such as osteoporosis

be active for your own reasons

Be active for fun, to spend time with family and friends, to accomplish a chore, to be fit, learn a new skill, sleep better, and relax. Being active out of a sense of guilt or obligation doesn't work in the long run.

I've found that in order to be consistent with physical activity I have to like what I'm doing... a lot. Experiment to find what activity is fun for you ... that's the only way you'll make the time and commitment to stick with it.

Lorna

The road ahead

map out your road to increasing your activity

Choose your activities and set your goals in the following chart. Keep track of your progress by noting your daily activity in your personal calendar.

DATE	MY ENDURANCE ACTIVITIES (AEROBIC)	GOAL DAYS/ WEEK	MY FLEXIBILITY ACTIVITIES	GOAL DAYS/ WEEK	MY STRENGTH ACTIVITIES	GOAL DAYS/ WEEK
	EXAMPLE: Walking	4	Yoga	3	Stair climbing	3

Refresh Your Life with Sleep

People need from six to nine hours of sleep per night. Pay attention to how much sleep you need to feel well rested. If you generally have a good sleep and yet do not wake up feeling rested, see your doctor.

"A good laugh and a long sleep are the best cures in the doctor's book. "

— IRISH PROVERB

Need a sleep tune-up?

Are you getting enough sleep? It may be time to consider ways to improve your sleep habits. Sleep is a basic necessity of life. Some researchers say that it allows your brain to replenish itself, absorb what you learned through the day and master new skills. When we sleep well, we wake up feeling refreshed, alert and ready to face daily challenges.

Reality Bites

drivers are asleep at the wheel

According to the Alberta Motor Association, 15 percent of drivers have reported falling asleep behind the wheel.

insomnia is common

75 percent of American adults experience a sleep problem at least a few nights a week. 39 percent get less than seven hours of sleep per night.

sleep is more difficult with age

One out of three adults 65 years and older complains of difficulty sleeping. Daytime naps and other lifestyle habits can interfere with nighttime sleep. The physical changes in our bodies as we age make sleep more difficult. However, sleep problems can also be due to medical and psychiatric conditions, so if you are experiencing persistent problems sleeping, talk to your doctor.

sleep has far reaching effects

Too little sleep can ruin your whole day. It can put jobs, relationships, productivity, health and safety at risk.

In the short-term, not enough sleep results in:

- tiredness
- irritability
- careless mistakes
- difficulty concentrating
- slower reaction times
- increased stress
- poor eating

In the long-term, not enough sleep may:

- lower metabolism and hormone production in a way that is similar to the effects of aging and the early stages of diabetes

"It is a common experience that a problem difficult at night is resolved in the morning after the committee of sleep has worked on it."

JOHN STEINBECK, AUTHOR

!

Many of these symptoms can be related to other medical conditions. See your doctor to discuss your concerns.

The only reasons to be in bed are:

- sleep
- sex
- sickness

"Sleep is the golden chain that ties our health and our bodies together."

THOMAS DEKKER, DRAMATIST

Keys to sleep

daytime habits

Exercise

A Stanford University Medical School study found that after 16 weeks in a moderate intensity exercise program, middle aged and older adults fell asleep about 15 minutes earlier and slept about 45 minutes longer at night.

Don't exercise just before bedtime if it interferes with your sleep.

Monitor napping

Avoid napping if it interferes with your sleep at night.

Less caffeine

Avoid caffeine after noon. Caffeine is commonly found in coffee, tea, colas and chocolate.

bedroom rules

Decorate your bedroom to achieve a relaxed, inviting atmosphere.

Move the TV out.

bedtime

Stick to a consistent bedtime.

Establish a relaxing and nurturing bedtime ritual such as drinking warm milk, reading, bathing by candlelight, relaxing to music, or applying cream to your feet.

Distract yourself. If you can't sleep after 20 minutes, get up and read or do some other relaxing activity, then try to fall asleep.

Although reading is commonly not recommended at bedtime, many people find it relaxing and enjoyable.

The road ahead

map out your road to recharging with sleep

Ask yourself:

- How many hours of sleep do I get on average?
- How many hours of sleep would I like to get each night?
- What would be a great bedtime ritual for me?
- What can I do to make my bedroom a more restful place?

Since I increased my sleep I'm more alert, calmer, and more productive. I've also cut my coffee consumption in half because I don't feel so tired in the morning.

Lorna

My answers:

"Whether you think you can or you can't, you're right."

HENRY FORD

Real Life Weight Loss Motivators:

Dad got Diabetes — I knew I could be next.

Kim, 32
Lost 32 lbs in 1 year

I was recommended to lose weight because of chronic back pain. Once I started losing - I just felt better and kept on losing.

Deb, 45
Lost 50 lbs in 2 years

I was getting older and had always been overweight. I didn't want to keep gaining and I wanted to look better.

Emily, 24
Lost 30 lbs in 1 year

Be a Healthy Weight

Need a weight tune-up?

read the Recharge Your Eating Habits and Revitalize Your Days with Activity sections

Healthy eating and daily activity are the foundations of a healthy weight.

use these two simple tools to tell if you're at a healthy weight

Waist measurement:

- As a Woman, you are considered overweight if you have a waist circumference of more than 35 inches (88 centimetres).
- As a Man, you are considered overweight if you have a waist circumference of more than 40 inches (102 centimetres).

Body Mass Index (BMI)

BMI is used to assess the risk of developing health problems based on body weight. The following BMI chart is intended for adults, except women who are pregnant or lactating.

NOTE: Age related BMI charts are available from Health Canada for children. (See the reference pages at the end of the journal for contact information)

Body Mass Index Chart (BMI) Chart

1) Find your height in the left-hand column labelled Height (in inches).

2) Move across to your Weight (in pounds).

3) The number at the top of the column is the BMI for that height and weight. *

For example, consider the highlighted numbers: a woman is 65 inches or 5 feet 5 inches and 148 pounds. Find 65 inches on the left hand column and move your finger across to 150 pounds (148 pounds rounded to the nearest number). Look at the top BMI row above the weight to see her BMI is 25. Find your BMI in this manner.

BMI	19	20	21	22	23	24	25	26	27	28	29	30	31	32	33	34	35
Height (inches)	Body Weight (pounds)																
58	91	96	100	105	110	115	119	124	129	134	138	143	148	153	158	162	167
59	94	99	104	109	114	119	124	128	133	138	143	148	153	158	163	168	173
60	97	102	107	112	118	123	128	133	138	143	148	153	158	163	168	174	179
61	100	106	111	116	122	127	132	137	143	148	153	158	164	169	174	180	185
62	104	109	115	120	126	131	136	142	147	153	158	164	169	175	180	186	191
63	107	113	118	124	130	135	141	146	152	158	163	169	175	180	186	191	197
64	110	116	122	128	134	140	145	151	157	163	169	174	180	186	192	197	204
65	114	120	126	132	138	144	150	156	162	168	174	180	186	192	198	204	210
66	118	124	130	136	142	148	155	161	167	173	179	186	192	198	204	210	216
67	121	127	134	140	146	153	159	166	172	178	185	191	198	204	211	217	223
68	125	131	138	144	151	158	164	171	177	184	190	197	203	210	216	223	230
69	128	135	142	149	155	162	169	176	182	189	196	203	209	216	223	230	236
70	132	139	146	153	160	167	174	181	188	195	202	209	216	222	229	236	243
71	136	143	150	157	165	172	179	186	193	200	208	215	222	229	236	243	250
72	140	147	154	162	169	177	184	191	199	206	213	221	228	235	242	250	258
73	144	151	159	166	174	182	189	197	204	212	219	227	235	242	250	257	265
74	148	155	163	171	179	186	194	202	210	218	225	233	241	249	256	264	272
75	152	160	168	176	184	192	200	208	216	224	232	240	248	256	264	272	279
76	156	164	172	180	189	197	205	213	221	230	238	246	254	263	271	279	287

*** If your BMI is below 19 or above 35** you will need to use this formula to calculate your BMI:

(your weight in kilograms) divided by (your height in meters X your height in meters)

For example, a man who weighs 104 kilograms and is 1.7 meters tall:
104 divided by (1.7 X 1.7) = 35.98 (round this number off) This man has a BMI of 36

What is your risk?

Weight Class	BMI	Risk of developing health problems
Underweight	Less than 18.5	Increased risk.
Normal Weight	18.5 to 24.9	Least risk
Overweight	25 or greater	Increased risk. Risk escalates as BMI rises. Extremely high risk when the BMI reaches 40 or higher.

As a dietitian, I could usually predict the success of people's weight loss effort from their attitude on their first visit. Those with many excuses and faint intentions would spin their wheels, while people who had initiated some changes on their own, were on their way to success.

Beverly

Reality Bites

short-term goals aren't the answer

Weight loss for occasions such as a graduation or wedding is usually temporary. When the occasion is over and you resume your usual intake or make up for the foods that you missed on your diet, the weight returns.

fad diets don't work for the long-term

Going on a diet is often a predictor of future weight gain. Seldom do diets teach you healthy eating for the long-term. However, in the short-term they make you much more aware of your food choices and decrease your calorie intake.

your weight affects your future health

Extra weight increases your risk of developing a number of chronic diseases including: Type 2 diabetes, high cholesterol, high blood pressure, heart disease, gallbladder disease, certain cancers, and sleep apnoea.

your body weight reflects your lifestyle

Everything from what you eat, your exercise habits to how you handle stress, helps to determine your weight. Healthy bodies come in a range of weights, shapes and sizes.

breakfast skippers weigh more

According to a study conducted in the United States, men and women who regularly skipped breakfast were four and a half times more likely to be obese as those who regularly ate breakfast.

more meals can be better

Having four or more meals per day has been shown to cut your obesity risk in half, even if you eat the same number of calories. Spreading the calories into four meals at regular times evens out the highs and lows of blood sugar that can affect appetite and fat storage.

portion sizes are growing

Today, a restaurant serving of spaghetti and meatballs is more than double the calories of a serving of spaghetti and meatballs twenty years ago while a bagel has increased by 210 calories in those twenty years. Today's larger food portions are a contributor to weight gain and risk of disease.

meals eaten out can have hidden calories

People who regularly eat breakfast or dinner in fast food outlets or restaurants are twice as likely to gain weight. These meals are generally higher in fat and the servings are larger.

> ***"The most powerful technology driving the obesity epidemic is television. The relationship is nearly as strong as what you see between smoking and lung cancer."***
>
> STEVEN GORTMAKER, HARVARD SCHOOL OF PUBLIC HEALTH

Ten-Pound Weight Loss Reduces Risk

Achieving a modest weight loss can improve overall health. A ten-pound weight loss for an overweight person can reduce the risk for Type 2 diabetes, heart disease and metabolic syndrome.

American Dietetic Association

Weight loss bonuses:

I feel less back pain and I am more energetic and self-confident after losing 15 pounds.

Cindy, 39

I am more flexible and have better self-esteem after losing 18 pounds.

Sherry, 49

What made the weight loss program work this time?

I realized eating wasn't making me fat - it was not eating for long periods of time and then eating too much of the wrong foods.

Rumina, 36

I never knew what a proper portion size was before I started Weight Watchers.

Emily, 24

I finally heard an eating maxim that made sense to me: eat what makes you feel good after you've eaten it.

Cindy, 39

Keys to weight loss

lose weight for your health and vitality

The weight loss keys are intended to improve your vitality and decrease your risk of chronic disease.

cure the root problem

If you eat in response to stress, fatigue or depression – treat these problems first. Learn how your feelings drive your eating by recording your intake of food for at least a week. You will be able to identify both your good and bad habits, including emotional triggers and temptations to overeat.

look for a long-term solution

Unfortunately, there's no magic pill here. The key to losing weight and keeping it off is simple healthy eating and regular activity.

set a goal

A committed decision to lose weight is the best predictor of success. Lose weight for your own reasons.

For motivation, find a picture of yourself when you looked and felt great and post it on your mirror or fridge.

make physical activity a priority

Physical activity is key to appetite control, maintaining muscle and long-term weight loss. Muscle uses more calories to maintain than fat. Muscle is also more compact; therefore, people who have increased their physical activity may see a change in their waist measurement or how their clothes fit before they see a change on the scale.

cook light and simple

Plan for simple healthy meals including at least three of the four food groups. Use a minimum amount of healthy fat in your cooking.

shop after you've eaten

Don't grocery shop when you're hungry, it can lead to impulse buying.

watch your serving size

Healthy servings are a key to a healthy weight. Use Canada's Food Guide or the Everyday Guide at right as a gauge to portion size. Don't assume serving sizes in restaurants are healthy for you.

don't skip meals

Skipping meals can lead to overeating and poor food choices later.

plan meals ahead

Have the right groceries to make healthy meals. Lack of planning can result in poor food choices such as fast or convenienence foods that are high in calories. Notice that the outside aisles of grocery stores tend to have the healthier items, while the convenience foods are on the inner isles.

slow down

Enjoying a relaxed meal can help you to eat less.

watch the beverages

Regular intake of soda pop or alcohol adds many empty calories. Although fruit juice is a healthy choice in moderation, it adds unnecessary calories when consumed in large quantities.

A few sources for healthy tasty recipes:

Magazines
Chatelaine
Prevention
Weight Watchers

Cookbooks
Looney Spoons
Crazy Plates
The Wellness Kitchen*

Guide to Nutrition in Foods:
Wellness Foods A to Z*

**Available online @ berkeleywellness.com*

Everyday Guide for servings sizes:

ONE SERVING	A HANDY GUIDE FOR SIZE
3 ounces meat, chicken or fish	A deck of cards
1 cup of vegetables	Your fist
$^1/_2$ cup of cooked pasta	Ice cream scoop
1 ounce of cheese	4 dice
1 cup dry cereal	A large handful
2 table-spoons of peanut butter	A golf ball
1 cup raw vegetables, yoghurt or fruit	Fits in an average woman's hand

!

If you lose more than five percent of your body weight without trying to, talk to your doctor. (For a 150-pound person, five percent would be seven and one-half pounds)

"The investment you make in yourself today will determine the quality of your life in the days and years to come."

AUTHOR UNKNOWN

"I look forward to being older, when what you look like becomes less and less an issue and what you are is the point."

SUSAN SARANDON, ACTRESS

limit restaurant eating

Choose a restaurant that has healthy options, moderate-serving sizes or will customize your order. Apply the same principles from the Recharge Your Eating Habits section when ordering in restaurants.

think about your food choices

When making food choices, eat what you know will make you feel good after you've eaten it.

don't rely only on your scale

Other key measures of progress towards a healthy weight include waist measurement, the fit of your clothes, your energy level and how you feel. Also, congratulate yourself for changes in your lifestyle such as healthy food choices, portion control, regular meals, and regular physical activity.

work through setbacks

Setbacks are normal. Don't beat yourself up! Learn what you can from each setback and get yourself back on track.

age well

As you age you need fewer calories to hold your weight. Avoid gaining weight by eating fewer calories. Keeping a healthy weight:

- Lowers your risk of heart disease, arthritis, cancer and other diseases.
- Helps to avoid developing problems with getting around and taking care of yourself.

The road ahead

map out your road to a healthy weight

Set a goal and review your progress every week. Set a modest goal and then set a new one when you reach that goal. A gradual weight loss of one to two pounds per week is safe for most people.

"Determine that the thing can and shall be done, and then we shall find the way."

ABRAHAM LINCOLN

MY GOAL	WHAT I NEED TO DO	TIME TO ACHIEVE	CHECK-UPS
EXAMPLE: Lose 10 pounds	Swim 4 days per week Take the stairs instead of the elevator Eat breakfast every day	3 months	Monthly weights and measurements

keep a food diary to find the root problem

In a notebook make the following headings:

FOOD OR DRINK	AMOUNT	TIME	PLACE	ALONE OR WITH SOMEONE	ACTIVITY	FEELINGS
EXAMPLE: Toast with peanut butter	1 tbsp peanut butter 1 slice bread	9:30 PM	family room	alone	watching TV	tired

Rethink Alcohol, Tobacco & Drugs

One Standard Drink equals:

Wine (12% alcohol)
5 ounces (142 mls)

Spirits
(40% alcohol)
1 $^{1}/_{2}$ ounces (43 mls)

Beer
(5 % alcohol)
12 ounces (341 mls)

Higher alcohol beers and coolers have more alcohol than one standard drink.

Reality Bites

using alcohol, tobacco and other drugs to cope

Turning to alcohol, tobacco or other drugs to avoid anxiety and sadness can be a hard habit to break. Drugs become the bandaid, but the root problem remains.

substance abuse affects people of all ages, income and education levels

- **Alcohol and tobacco** are the most widely abused substances by young people and adults.
- **Illegal drug use** is the most common among adolescents and young adults. Street drugs are likely to be hazardous and their effects unpredictable. These drugs can cause serious problems no matter how often or when they are taken.
- Overuse of **medicine to sleep or for anxiety** is the most common among seniors. Prescription drugs are generally considered safe when used as prescribed. However, overuse of drugs such as painkillers and anti-anxiety drugs can lead to dependence.

"If you want to be happy, put your effort into controlling the sail, not the wind."

ANONYMOUS

Reality Bites - Alcohol

low risk drinking guidelines (LRDG)

Drink no more than two standard drinks per day.

Limit your weekly intake to 14 or fewer standard drinks for men, nine or fewer for women. Spread these drinks out through the week. Drinking your weekly limit in one sitting can be hazardous to your health. It takes less alcohol to affect women than men because women are generally smaller and their bodies contain less water to dilute alcohol. Women also burn alcohol more slowly than men.

Here are some tips to avoid getting drunk: drink slowly and make a drink last at least an hour, take alcohol with food and drink non-alcoholic beverages.

(The LRDG are from the Centre for Addiction and Mental Health & the University of Toronto. The LRDG are for healthy people of legal drinking age. However, there are groups and situations when drinking is inadvisable - e.g., pregnancy, addiction, chronic illness, safety).

alcohol has both positive and negative effects

Alcohol's protective effect on the heart has received a lot of press. However, alcohol's protective effect can be achieved with as little as one drink every other day. For most people, having more than two drinks a day does more harm than good. Drinking more than recommended increases risk of injuries and certain chronic diseases such as stroke, heart disease, diabetes, osteoporosis, and some types of cancers. Discuss the pros and cons of alcohol intake with your doctor.

It is estimated that one out of seven North Americans abuse or are dependent on alcohol.

!

You are abusing alcohol if:

- it interferes with work, home or school
- you drink and drive
- you have had legal problems because of it
- it has negatively affected personal relationships

Health Canada

Smoking is a greater cause of death and disability than any single disease.

World Health Organization

Teens are leading the way

Smoking has dramatically decreased among 15 to 19 year olds. In 1999, 28 percent of teens were smoking. In 2003, only 18 percent were smoking. For the first time in nearly a decade teens were smoking less than adults!

Health Canada

Reality Bites - Smoking

smoking makes people sick

Smoking increases a person's risk of developing lung cancer, heart disease, stroke, mouth disease, bronchitis and emphysema, and impotence.

Canadians are quitting

Health Canada Surveys have shown 35 percent of Canadians were smoking in 1985. In 2003 approximately 21 percent of Canadians were smoking.

In 1985, daily smokers consumed around 21 cigarettes per day. In 2003, daily smokers consumed around 16 cigarettes per day.

renew your body by quitting

Here are some of the improvements you can look forward to when you quit smoking:

- in eight hours your oxygen increases to a normal level
- in two days your sense of smell and taste return
- in two weeks to three months your circulation improves and your lungs work 30% better
- in one year your risk of heart attack is cut in half
- in 15 years your risk of heart attack is that of a non-smoker

Keys to dealing with your dependence

take personal responsibility

Acknowledge that you have a problem and decide to quit.

seek help

Counselling and support groups are very helpful, as people tend to abuse substances as a method of coping with other problems. Counselling will help you to:

- determine what real problems the substance is masking
- learn new ways to cope
- identify high risk situations
- design a healthier lifestyle
- identify a support system
- build confidence and motivation

Discuss your dependency with your doctor and ask for advice and support programs.

Access your provincial addictions program.

The road ahead

Plan to take back the control over your life.

- Acknowledge if you have a dependency and seek help.
- Acknowledge what purpose the dependency serves in your life.
- Make your plan to quit.
- Ensure you have support for your plan.

"The two important things I did learn were that you are as powerful and strong as you allow yourself to be, and that the most difficult part of any endeavour is taking the first step, making the first decision."

ROBYN DAVIDSON, AUTHOR OF TRACKS - A STORY OF HER 1700-MILE SOLO TREK ON FOOT ACROSS THE AUSTRALIAN OUTBACK

My notes:

"Believe in the possibility you can."

CELESTE NEEDHAM, YOGA INSTRUCTOR

Vitality Rating Scale

The Vitality Rating Scale will help you to measure how your personal choices affect your vitality. Rate yourself on a scale of 0 to 5 on each of the statements. Base your answers on your lifestyle over the last month. Use your results to consider opportunities to energize your lifestyle.

Never	Rarely	Sometimes	About half the time	Frequently	Almost Always
0	1	2	3	4	5

DATE:										
BALANCE	**SCORE (0-5)**									
The choices I make every day reflect my priorities and values.										
I manage my time so I accomplish what I truly want, feeling satisfied and proud. I don't over commit.										
I foster inner growth and spirituality.										
I make a conscious effort to remove clutter from my life.										
I surround myself only with people who give me energy.										
BALANCE TOTAL /25										

DATE:										
EATING HABITS	**SCORE (0-5)**									
I choose at least 3 servings of whole grain products every day.										
I eat 5 or more servings of fruits and/or vegetables every day.										
I use healthy fats such as oils, soft margarines, nuts, seeds and fish.										
I drink milk, eat milk products daily or take a calcium supplement that provides for the needs of my age group. (see p. 20)										
I choose lean meats, fish, eggs, beans or lentils as protein sources daily.										
EATING HABITS TOTAL /25										

ACTIVITY	**SCORE (0-5)**									
I am active for at least 30 minutes most days of the week.										
I do activities that build muscle in my arms, mid-section and legs at least 2 days a week.										
I do stretching (flexibility) activities at least 4 days a week.										
I do activities that strengthen my heart (aerobic activities) at least 4 days a week.										
Activity is included in my daily routines.										
ACTIVITY TOTAL /25										

Never	Rarely	Sometimes	About half the time	Frequently	Almost Always
0	1	2	3	4	5

DATE:										
SLEEP	**SCORE (0-5)**									
I get enough sleep most nights.										
My bedroom is a restful place.										
I am able to concentrate and perform tasks well because I get enough sleep.										
I keep alert during the day without depending on caffeine or other stimulants.										
I follow a relaxing bedtime routine.										
SLEEP TOTAL /25										

WEIGHT	**SCORE (0-5)**									
My weight is in the healthy range of the Body Mass Index. (See BMI Chart p. 33)										
My waist is 35 inches (88 cm) or less for women and 40 inches (102 cm) or less for men.										
I plan regular meals starting my day with a good breakfast.										
My serving sizes contribute to a healthy weight.										
Physical activity is a priority.										
WEIGHT TOTAL /25										

DATE:										
ALCOHOL, TOBACCO, DRUGS	**SCORE (0-5)**									
I am a non-smoker.										
I drink moderately or not at all: (Women this is 9 or fewer drinks a week. Men this is 14 or fewer drinks a week).										
I cope without relying on drugs or alcohol.										
I choose not to drink & drive.										
My family & work life are free from the interference of alcohol & drugs.										
ALCOHOL, TOBACCO, DRUGS TOTAL /25										

Your results

Tally your scores to see where you're at now and then measure your progress over time. For each section the highest possible score is 25.

- **A score of 0 to 10: Needs serious work**
- **A score of 11 to 15: Room for improvement**
- **A score of 16 to 20: Starting to look and feel good**
- **A score of 21 to 25: Looking and feeling great**

Looking at the whole picture

Write your total from each section in the chart below.

DATE:										
VITALITY SCORE	**SCORE (0-25)**									
Balance										
Eating Habits										
Activity										
Sleep										
Weight										
Alcohol, Tobacco, Drugs										
VITALITY TOTAL /150										

"Twenty years from now you will be more disappointed by the things that you didn't do than by the ones you did do. So throw off the bowlines. Sail away from the safe harbor. Catch the trade winds in your sails. Explore. Dream. Discover."

MARK TWAIN

Life situations throw us curve balls that change our life balance. For example, physical activity may be the first to go when work piles up, which is when we need it most because activity helps us to think clearer and be more productive. Be an observer in your life and notice what helps you to find balance.

Decide which areas of your vitality are your priorities right now. You might choose the areas where you scored the lowest, or maybe the areas where you think you can make the most impact right now. Think about what it would take to move you to the next level. Map out your plan using the Road Ahead part of the Vitality Section(s) you choose to work on. Recheck your progress every three to six months.

Vitals

"The chief condition on which life, health and vigor depend on, is action. It is by action that an organism develops its faculties, increases its energy, and attains the fulfillment of its destiny."

COLIN POWELL,
U.S. SECRETARY OF STATE 2001 TO 2005

What are Vitals?

Every year in your birthday month ensure your records are complete. Review your Vitality Rating Scale and your Vitals, and then make your goals for the upcoming months.

Vitals are the details of your health. This Vitals section helps you to monitor your health and be more mindful of it. You are prompted to document your:

- **Health History**

  An accurate history can help your doctor to recognize risks, make diagnoses and recommend treatments.

- **Screening Tests & Vaccinations**

  Screening tests can catch disease early. Vaccinations help to prevent disease.

- **Dental, Eye & Hearing Health**

  Learn to protect your senses and catch problems early.

- **Appointments & Symptoms**

  Record changes in your health and discuss them with your doctor.

Studies have shown that good communication between a doctor and patient results in:

- better control of headaches
- better control of asthma
- better test results such as blood pressure or blood sugar
- better control of cancer pain and dental pain
- better control of depression
- less anxiety

• Medicines, Vitamins & Other Treatments

Every treatment can affect your health and interact with other treatments. Note how the treatment works for you and share the information with your doctor.

• Planning for the Unexpected & People

Protect your health and finances in the event you are not able to communicate your wishes. Write down contact information of your family, friends and health care team.

• Notes & Resources

Jot down notes and see where you can go for more information.

The time that you spend filling in the journal is a great personal investment. Keep your journal accurate and up-to-date. Take the journal to medical appointments so you can fill in test results and to be sure your concerns are addressed. You are the best advocate for your own health!

Health History

Doctors collect their patients' family histories to determine if they have family tendencies to heart disease, stroke, cancer and other conditions. This knowledge helps doctors to determine which tests should be ordered and what advice to give their patients.

Family Health History

Record any major illnesses or chronic diseases of your brothers, sisters, parents, aunts, uncles and grandparents. Knowledge of family health will help you and your children to prevent conditions or seek early treatment. It also gives your doctor a better understanding of your health risks.

Family Health History

RELATIVE	DIAGNOSIS	AGE AT DIAGNOSIS	COMMENTS AND UPDATES (INCLUDING CAUSE OF DEATH IF DECEASED)

Update this record each year before your annual exam.

"I think of a hero as someone who understands the degree of responsibility that comes with his freedom."

BOB DYLAN

RELATIVE	DIAGNOSIS	AGE AT DIAGNOSIS	COMMENTS AND UPDATES (INCLUDING CAUSE OF DEATH IF DECEASED)

When people are more involved in their medical appointments they:

- feel more in control of their health
- take more initiative to make changes
- recall information better
- attend follow-up appointments
- have better results

My Diagnoses

Note your diagnoses. Women also note your pregnancies and whether you had any complications such as gestational diabetes or RH incompatibility.

My Blood Type is ___________

DATE	DIAGNOSIS	DOCTOR	TREATMENT

A good medical appointment should bring out information from your point of view including health concerns, preferences, and expectations.

DATE	DIAGNOSIS	DOCTOR	TREATMENT

My Emergency Room Visits & Hospital Stays

If you received a tetanus vaccination while in emergency or in a hospital be sure to include it in your vaccination record.

DATE	REASON	HOSPITAL	TREATMENT

Your participation in discussing treatment alternatives leads to treatment decisions that best meet your needs and preferences.

DATE	REASON	HOSPITAL	TREATMENT

My Surgeries & Procedures

DATE	SURGERY OR PROCEDURE	HOSPITAL	DOCTOR

!

Aspirin should NOT be taken before surgery, as it can increase your risk of bleeding. **Vitamin E, certain herbs (e.g., Gingko) and other over-the-counter medicines** can also increase your risk of bleeding. Check with your surgeon to find out how long before surgery you should avoid taking these medicines.

"I've felt that the only way to survive was with dignity, pride and courage."

ERIC CLAPTON

DATE	SURGERY OR PROCEDURE	HOSPITAL	DOCTOR

Weight & Measurements

Take your weight and measurements at the same time of day and with the same equipment. Don't weigh yourself daily, especially if you are trying to lose weight, allow time for change. Discuss any questions about your progress with a health professional.

	GOALS	DATE	DATE	DATE	DATE	DATE	DATE	DATE	DATE
HEIGHT									
WEIGHT									
BMI*									
WAIST									
HIPS									
CLOTHING SIZE									

* *See BMI chart on page 33.*

After whether you smoke or not, weight is the most important measure of health.

— Dr Walter Willett, Eat, Drink & Be Healthy, 2001

	GOALS	DATE	DATE	DATE	DATE	DATE	DATE	DATE	DATE
HEIGHT									
WEIGHT									
BMI*									
WAIST									
HIPS									
CLOTH-ING SIZE									

	GOALS	DATE	DATE	DATE	DATE	DATE	DATE	DATE	DATE
HEIGHT									
WEIGHT									
BMI*									
WAIST									
HIPS									
CLOTH-ING SIZE									

!

Everyone loses a little height with normal aging. But a significant loss of 4 centimetres (1 1/2 inches) or greater OR more than 2 centimetres in one year (3/4 inch) — may be one of the earliest signs of osteoporosis.

Osteoporosis Society of Canada

"If you can dream it, you can do it."

WALT DISNEY

Screening Tests & Vaccinations

Screening Tests

Screening tests have been designed to catch disease at an early stage, so it can be treated more effectively. Some of these tests are routinely recommended at annual physical exams while others depend on your personal risk for a condition or disease.

<table>
<tr><th>SCREENING FOR:</th><th>AGES 18 TO 39</th><th>AGES 40 TO 49</th><th>AGES 50 TO 64</th><th>AGE 65 & OLDER</th></tr>
<tr><td rowspan="1">High Blood Pressure
Uncontrolled high blood pressure can lead to heart disease, stroke and kidney disease.</td><td colspan="4">Screening Recommended by Health Canada
• Starting at age 21, blood pressure should be checked at least every two years.
• Blood pressure should be checked every year if it is high normal (130/85 to 135/89).
• If blood pressure is high (140/90 or higher) your doctor will recommend you have it checked more often.</td></tr>
<tr><td rowspan="4">High Cholesterol
High cholesterol levels can lead to heart disease or heart attack.</td><td colspan="4">Screening Recommended by the Working Group on Hypercholesterolemia and other Dyslipidemias (Canadian)</td></tr>
<tr><td></td><td></td><td colspan="2">• Women who are post menopausal or over 50 should have their cholesterol checked.</td></tr>
<tr><td></td><td colspan="3">• Men over 40 should have their cholesterol checked.</td></tr>
<tr><td colspan="4">• In addition, people of any age with diabetes, high blood pressure, smoking, abdominal obesity, a family history of premature heart disease, or symptoms of hardening of the arteries should have their cholesterol checked. Ask your family doctor when and how often you should have your cholesterol checked and what levels are ideal for you.</td></tr>
</table>

PLEASE NOTE:

Your doctor may recommend more frequent, earlier, or additional screening based on your personal risk factors and symptoms. Recommendations may change over time, so use this list as a guide and check with your doctor. The guidelines are current as of February 2005.

SCREENING FOR:	AGES 18 TO 39	AGES 40 TO 49	AGES 50 TO 64	AGE 65 & OLDER
Diabetes	**Screening Recommended by the Canadian Diabetes Association**			
Diabetes can lead to poor circulation, eye disease, heart disease and kidney disease.		• Screening for diabetes using a simple blood sugar test should be performed every three years in people 40 years of age and older. A fasting blood sugar of 6.1 mmol/L and higher is abnormal.		
Metabolic Syndrome	**Screening Recommended by the Working Group on Hypercholesterolemia and other Dyslipidemias (Canadian)**			
Metabolic syndrome is a cluster of health risks that greatly increases your chance of developing **heart disease, stroke,** and **diabetes**. At least one quarter of Canadians has this syndrome.		Screening for metabolic syndrome should be performed after age 50 or after menopause for women. Men should be screened after age 40. You are diagnosed with metabolic syndrome if you have **three or more** of the following: • Abdominal obesity - a waist circumference of more than For women: 88 centimetres (35 inches) For men: 102 centimetres (40 inches) • Triglycerides (a blood fat) of 1.7 mmol/L or greater • HDL cholesterol (good cholesterol) For women: less than 1.3 mmol/L For men: less than 1.0 mmol/L • A blood pressure of 130/85 or higher • A fasting blood sugar of 6.2 - 7.0 mmol/L Metabolic Syndrome is also called Syndrome X, Insulin Resistance Syndrome, and Dysmetabolic Syndrome.		

Screening Tests, continued

SCREENING FOR:	AGES 18 TO 39	AGES 40 TO 49	AGES 50 TO 64	AGE 65 & OLDER
Changes in Vision and Eye Diseases Vision problems do not always produce symptoms.	**Screening Recommended by the Canadian Association of Optometrists** • General Recommendation for a vision exam: Adults 20-64 years of age - every one to two years. • Your doctor or optometrist may recommend vision exams more often.			• Vision exam every year at age 65 and older.
Tooth decay and gum disease The goal of the six-month check-up is to catch problems early.	**Screening Recommended by the Canadian Dental Association** • Dental checkups every six months.			
Hearing Loss Hearing loss starts gradually and can often go unnoticed.	**Screening Recommended by the Canadian Association of Speech - Language Pathologists & Audiologists** • If you suspect you have a hearing problem see your doctor or an audiologist.			
Osteoporosis Osteoporosis can lead to broken bones and back pain.	**Screening Recommended by the Osteoporosis Society of Canada** • Bone density exam may be recommended at any age for high-risk individuals. Ask your doctor if you are at high risk.			
				• Bone density exam for men and women at age 65 and older.

SCREENING FOR:	AGES 18 TO 39	AGES 40 TO 49	AGES 50 TO 64	AGE 65 & OLDER
Colorectal Cancer Colon and rectal cancers are the third most common cancers in Canada.			**Screening Recommended by the Canadian Cancer Society** • Stool sample at least every two years starting at the age of 50. Your doctor may also recommend sigmoidoscopy and colonoscopy. Those who are at higher than average risk of developing colorectal cancer should discuss an individual plan of surveillance with their doctor.	
Skin Cancer Learn what to look for, and check your skin regularly, as most skin cancers can be cured if they're caught early.	**Screening Recommended by the Canadian Cancer Society** See your doctor if you notice any of the following: • A birthmark or a mole that changes shape, colour, size or surface • Any new growth on your skin - pale, pearly nodules that may grow larger and crust, or red scaly, sharply defined patches • Any sore that doesn't heal • Any patch of skin that bleeds, oozes, swells, itches or becomes red and bumpy			
Cervical Cancer (Women only) Most cases of cervical cancer occur in women who have either never had a Pap test or have not had one recently.	**Screening Recommended by the Canadian Cancer Society** • Women who become sexually active should have a Pap test and pelvic examination every 1 to 3 years depending on the screening guidelines in their province. Even if you have stopped having sex, you should continue to have the tests. Using a condom during sex decreases the chance that you will pick up human papilloma virus (HPV), which is a risk factor for cervical cancer.			

Screening Tests, continued

SCREENING FOR:	AGES 18 TO 39	AGES 40 TO 49	AGES 50 TO 64	AGE 65 & OLDER
Breast Cancer (Women only) One in nine women will develop breast cancer in her lifetime. Survival is much higher when cancer is found at an earlier stage.	**Screening Recommended by the Canadian Cancer Society** Women over the age of 20 should perform monthly breast self-exams and report any changes to their doctor.			
	• Women from 20-39 years should have a breast exam by a trained professional every year.	• Women aged 40 and over should have a breast exam by a trained professional at least every two years.	• Women between 50 and 69 years of age should have a screening mammogram (a breast cancer screening x-ray) at least once every two years. If you are under age 50 or over 69 and are at a higher risk for breast cancer, you should discuss with your doctor when mammography may be appropriate for you.	
Prostate Cancer (Men only) Prostate cancer is strongly linked with increasing age.	**Screening Recommended by the Canadian Cancer Society**			
			• All men over the age of 50 years should discuss with their doctor the potential benefits and risks of early detection of prostate cancer using Prostate Specific Antigen (PSA) and digital rectal examinations (DRE). The PSA test is not used as routinely as it once was.	
	• Men at higher risk because of family history or those of African ancestry should discuss the need for testing at an earlier age.			

Nearly one in four Canadians has high blood pressure. Almost half of these people are unaware they have high blood pressure.

Canadian Heart Health Surveys 1986-1992

Blood pressure lifestyle tips:

- be at a healthy weight
- include fruits, vegetables and low fat dairy products daily
- limit alcohol intake
- be physically active
- limit the use of salt

Blood Pressure

My target blood pressure range (discuss with your doctor):

____

A diagnosis of high blood pressure usually takes three appointments. Two blood pressure checks are taken at each appointment.

DATE	BP	DATE	BP	DATE	BP

A healthy lifestyle is the newest drug

CANADIAN HYPERTENSION EDUCATION PROGRAM RECOMMENDATIONS, 2005

Before having your blood pressure measured:

- make sure you have been out of the cold for an hour
- avoid caffeine and smoking for 30 minutes
- avoid alcohol for at least 8 hours
- avoid heavy physical activity for 2 hours
- empty your bowel and bladder

The Canadian Hypertension Society

Blood Pressure, continued

DATE	BP	DATE	BP	DATE	BP	DATE	BP

Blood Cholesterol

Your doctor may measure your total cholesterol level first. If your total level is high, a second test may be done. The second test will be after a 12-14 hour fast. During the fast you should drink water. The second test will usually measure HDL cholesterol (good), LDL cholesterol (bad), and triglycerides (another form of blood fat). Ask your doctor for your target levels.

DATE	TOTAL CHOLESTEROL	HDL CHOLESTEROL	LDL CHOLESTEROL	TOTAL / HDL CHOLESTEROL RATIO	TRIGLYCERIDES
TARGET LEVELS					

Four out of 10 Canadian men and women have cholesterol levels above the desirable range.

Heart & Stroke Foundation of Canada

Cholesterol lifestyle tips:

- be at a healthy weight
- be physically active
- choose healthy fats
- eat soluble fibre daily

Blood Sugar

60,000 Canadians were diagnosed with diabetes in 2003.

If you are at a higher risk for developing diabetes, you can lower your risk by 58 percent if you lose 10 pounds and walk 30 minutes a day

Diabetes Prevention Program Research Group, NIH

DATE	BLOOD SUGAR	FASTING OR TWO HOURS AFTER EATING

DATE	BLOOD SUGAR	FASTING OR TWO HOURS AFTER EATING

Haemoglobin A1C (HbA1C) is a blood test of the average blood sugar over the past 2 to 3 months. (measured in people who have diabetes)

DATE	HbA1C	DATE	HbA1C	DATE	HbA1C

Osteoporosis

One in four women over the age of 50 has osteoporosis. One in eight men over 50 also has the disease. However, the disease can strike at any age.

Osteoporosis Society of Canada

Adequate calcium intake accompanied by Vitamin D can slow the bone loss of aging. Weight bearing activities such as walking, and dancing help to build bone. If you have osteoporosis, your doctor may recommend medicine in addition to lifestyle changes.

Osteoporosis Society of Canada

	BONE DENSITY EXAM			NORMAL, OR OSTEO-POROSIS?
DATE	SITE	T SCORE	Z SCORE	
	HIP			
	SPINE			
	FOREARM			

DATE	SITE	T SCORE	Z SCORE	
	HIP			
	SPINE			
	FOREARM			

DATE	SITE	T SCORE	Z SCORE	
	HIP			
	SPINE			
	FOREARM			

Vitamin D 'The Sunshine Vitamin'

Unlike other vitamins, Vitamin D isn't absorbed from many foods. Vitamin D is mostly found in cold water fish & fortified milk. Most Vitamin D comes from the sun reacting with your skin. In Canada, it's often necessary to take Vitamin D supplements in the winter.

! Eating habits account for about 30 percent of all cancers in western countries.

The World Health Organization

+ **To lower your risk for cancer:**

- Eat 5 to 10 servings of vegetables & fruit each day
- Eat high fibre and lower fat foods
- Limit your alcohol intake to 1 to 2 drinks per day

Canadian Cancer Society

Cancer Checks — Men & Women

STOOL TEST	
DATE	RESULT

SIGMOIDOSCOPY	
DATE	RESULT

COLONOSCOPY	
DATE	RESULT

Cancer Checks — Women Only

PAP TEST					
DATE	RESULT	DATE	RESULT	DATE	RESULT

Regular physical activity has been shown to have a protective effect in reducing the risk of breast and colorectal cancer.

The World Health Organization

Breast self - exam: Mark monthly on your calendar

MAMMOGRAM

DATE	RESULT	DATE	RESULT

BREAST EXAM – DOCTOR

DATE	RESULT	DATE	RESULT

Cancer Checks — Men Only

Prostate cancer is the number one threat to Canadian men. It will afflict 1 in 8 men in their lifetime, 19,000 in 2005.

Prostate Cancer Research Foundation of Canada

PROSTATE EXAM (DRE) DIGITAL RECTAL EXAM

DATE	RESULT	DATE	RESULT

PSA TEST (BLOOD TEST)

DATE	RESULT	DATE	RESULT	DATE	RESULT

Other Tests

"They say that time changes things, but you actually have to change them yourself."

ANDY WARHOL

TEST	DATE	RESULT

Other Tests, continued

TEST	DATE	RESULT	DATE	RESULT	DATE	RESULT

Vaccinations

ADULT VACCINATIONS RECOMMENDED BY HEALTH CANADA	WHO NEEDS THIS VACCINE?	HOW OFTEN?	DATE
Diphtheria Diphtheria is an infection caused by bacteria that most often infect the nose or throat. Diptheria is a severe disease.	All adults	Every 10 years	
Tetanus Tetanus is a disease caused by a toxin (or poison) that blocks normal control of nerve reflexes in the spinal column. It is also called lockjaw.	All adults	Every 10 years	
(Tetanus and Diphtheria are usually given in one shot.)			
Measles A viral infection that results in high fever, runny nose, cough, inflammation of the eyelid and a rash. It can damage many parts of the body	All adults born in 1970 or later who are susceptible to measles.	Two doses total	
Mumps A viral infection that can cause fever, headache and swelling of the glands around the jaw and cheeks. It can go on to affect other parts of the body.	Adults born in 1970 or later with no history of mumps.	Two doses total	

The chart lists routine adult vaccinations (also called immunizations). Review your vaccination record with your doctor.

A 1996 survey of Quebec adults found that only 33 per cent had been vaccinated against tetanus in the previous 10 years.

ADULT VACCINATIONS RECOMMENDED BY HEALTH CANADA	WHO NEEDS THIS VACCINE?	HOW OFTEN?	DATE
Rubella Commonly known as German measles, is a viral infection that primarily affects the skin and lymph nodes, and can be serious in pregnant women.	Adolescent girls and women of childbearing age and health care workers.	Two doses total	
MMR (Measles, Mumps and Rubella are usually given in one shot.)			
Flu Shot (Influenza) Influenza is a contagious disease that is caused by the influenza virus.	People 65 and older, and younger people at high risk for complications of the flu. Ask your doctor.	Every year	
Pneumococcal Pneumococcal diseases are bacterial infections of the lungs (pneumonia), the bloodstream (bacteraemia) and the the brain (encephalitis).	People 65 and older at high risk, and others at high risk for complications of pneumonia.	One dose	
Chickenpox A viral infection that starts with a fever and is followed by a rash of red spots that may be itchy.	Adults who have not had chickenpox.	One dose	
Hepatitis B A viral infection that causes Hepatitis. Passed on through infected blood or body fluids.	Universally recommended for Canadian adults.	A series of 3 doses (May vary)	

Diseases such as measles, polio, and diphtheria have almost disappeared in Canada and throughout the world as a direct result of immunization programs.

Canadian Coalition for Immunization Awareness and Promotion

The most effective way to protect yourself from the flu is to be vaccinated each year in the fall. Regular hand washing is another way to minimize your risk.

Travel Vaccinations

Traveling?

See your doctor or travel clinic 2 to 3 months before travel to allow time for vaccinations to be completed.

VACCINATIONS THAT MAY BE REQUIRED FOR TRAVEL TO CERTAIN COUNTRIES — CHECK WITH YOUR DOCTOR	WHO NEEDS THIS VACCINE?	HOW OFTEN?	DATE
Hepatitis A A viral infection that causes Hepatitis. Passed on through direct contact with infected people or through contaminated water or foods, especially shellfish. Hepatitis A and B vaccines are also available in one shot.	Travellers to high-risk areas. People at high risk because of their lifestyle, occupation or living conditions.	Should last 20 years. May require boosters	
Poliomyelitis (Polio) A viral infection that varies in severity from a mild illness with fever, to swelling of the lining of the brain, to paralysis and sometimes death.	Adults who have not been vaccinated or who have not had a booster shot in the past 10 years, and are travelling to high-risk countries.	3 doses	
Yellow fever A viral disease spread by a mosquito bite that starts with a fever, chills, headache, generalized muscle pain, severe fatigue, nausea and vomiting and then progresses to a more serious illness.	For travellers going to many areas of Africa and South America.	Every 10 years	

For current travel information from the Government of Canada go to www.travelhealth.gc.ca

100 years ago, infectious diseases were the leading cause of death worldwide. Now, thanks to immunization programs, they cause less than 5% of all deaths in Canada.

Many infectious diseases have been controlled, but could return if immunization is not maintained.

The Value of Immunization in the Future of Canada's Health System.

VACCINATIONS THAT MAY BE REQUIRED FOR TRAVEL TO CERTAIN COUNTRIES — CHECK WITH YOUR DOCTOR	WHO NEEDS THIS VACCINE?	HOW OFTEN?	DATE
Meningococcal Disease A rare, but potentially fatal bacterial infection. The disease results in swelling of the brain and spinal cord or a bacterial infection in the blood.	Travellers going to high-risk areas.	No set schedule for boosters	
Typhoid A bacterial infection that causes serious illness.	Travellers to any country with under-developed water treatment systems and sanitation, particularly when travel is off tourist routes or involves budget accommodations.	Booster doses every 3 years	
Japanese encephalitis A viral infection that is transmitted by a mosquito bite. It causes a swelling of the brain and spinal cord that can lead to permanent nerve damage or death.	Travellers going to any area prone to Japanese encephalitis for more than 4 weeks.	No set schedule for boosters	
Rabies A serious viral infection that if untreated usually results in death.	Travellers planning extended visits to countries where rabies is widespread. A post-exposure vaccine exists for use following a bite by a rabid animal.	No set schedule for boosters	

Other Vaccinations

With the exception of clean drinking water, no other human invention has had the impact of vaccinations in reducing infectious diseases, not even antibiotics.

Canadian Coalition for Immunization Awareness and Prevention

OTHER VACCINATIONS	WHY I NEED IT	HOW OFTEN?	DATE

Dental, Eye & Hearing Health

Dental

Dental Care

Dental health is very important to your overall wellbeing. Research has identified a possible link between oral disease and other health problems such as diabetes, heart disease and stroke as well as pre-term and low birth-weight babies.

Preventative care is important to preserving the health of your mouth and teeth. The Canadian Dental Association recommends the following practices to maintain oral health.

Eat

- A healthy balanced diet for good dental health
- Limit between meal snacks

Brush

- To remove bacteria, and to prevent tooth decay and gum disease
- Brush for two to three minutes
- Ideally you should brush after every meal
- Replace your toothbrush every three months

Nine out of 10 Canadians will develop gum disease (gingivitis). Gums may become red, infected, puffy, and bleed with brushing.

To Prevent Gingivitis:

Brush twice a day and floss at least once a day. An essential-oil containing mouth rinse, such as Listerine, may also help to fight gingivitis.

"Always bear in mind that your own resolution to succeed is more important than any other one thing."

ABRAHAM LINCOLN

Floss

- To remove plaque on the one-third of your tooth that your brush does not reach
- Floss at least once a day

See your dentist

- For preventative check ups and professional cleaning

Check your gums

- Red, puffy, tender gums: gums that bleed easily or persistent bad breath are all reasons to visit your dentist

Dental Care

DATE	DENTIST	WORK DONE

Dental Check-ups, continued

Most tooth decay and gum disease can be prevented through proper care of teeth and gums.

Generally the best time to floss is after your last meal of the day.

DATE	DENTIST	WORK DONE

DATE	DENTIST	WORK DONE

Dental Appliances

Dental Appliances have been used to treat:

- grinding of the teeth
- jaw problems
- snoring
- obstructive sleep apnoea

BRACES / BITE GUARD / DENTURES / PARTIALS / ETC.	DENTIST	NOTES (DATE OF PRESCRIPTIONS, ETC.)

Dental Insurance Coverage

INSURANCE COMPANY	WHAT'S COVERED	PERCENT COVERED	HOW OFTEN	CLAIMS

Eye

Eye

Your eyes may not give you any warning that they require attention; therefore, regular check ups are important. Eighteen and 19 year olds should have annual eye exams. Adults 20 to 64 years old should have their eyes checked every one to two years. Those 65 years and older should have an eye exam every year. To keep your eyes healthy:

- Wear sunglasses that block 99 percent or 100 percent of ultraviolet (UV) rays (check the label). Exposure to UV light can contribute to the development of cataracts and macular degeneration (Canadian Optometrists Association). Take care not to scratch the lens of your sunglasses - they lose some of their protective effect.
- Ensure you have good lighting in your work area.
- Wear protective eyewear when playing sports.
- Wear safety equipment when handling chemicals or power tools.
- Be alert for symptoms of vision problems: headaches, nausea, tired or burning eyes, blurred vision, difficulty reading reports or newspapers.

On average we blink 12 times per minute. But we only blink 5 times per minute when we're on the computer, which can result in dry eyes. Remember to blink more often when you're on the computer. Relieve the discomfort by using artificial teardrops or gels.

Canadian Optometrists Association

Eye Appointments

An eye exam is often where symptoms of conditions and diseases such as high blood pressure and diabetes are first noted, making early treatment possible.

DATE	EYE DOCTOR	COMMENTS

! Adults at higher risk for eye problems may need eye exams more often. This includes those with diabetes, high blood pressure, or a family history of glaucoma. If your work is visually demanding or you are on medicine that may affect your eyes, you may also be required to have more frequent eye exams.

Canadian Optometrists Association

16 million Canadians wear prescription glasses.

Eyewear Industry Report

Eye Wear

DATE	GLASSES / CONTACTS	RIGHT EYE (OD)					LEFT EYE (OS)				
		POWER	CYL	AXIS	PRISM	ADD	POWER	CYL	AXIS	PRISM	ADD

"It is impossible for a man to learn what he thinks he already knows."

EPICTETUS, PHILOSOPHER

Eye Insurance Coverage

INSURANCE COMPANY	WHAT'S COVERED	PERCENT COVERED	HOW OFTEN	CLAIMS

Hearing

Hearing Care

Learn how to protect your hearing so it will last a lifetime. Recognize the symptoms of hearing loss so you can receive early treatment. The American Hearing Aid Associates lists the following symptoms of hearing loss:

- Trouble understanding speech that originates far away, such as in concert halls, theatres, or churches
- Difficulty hearing a phone ring
- Difficulty hearing when in a group of people or in the presence of background noise, such as traffic
- Avoiding social gatherings and other public occasions where you might feel embarrassed about misunderstanding others
- Asking others to repeat themselves because you have trouble understanding what is being said
- Turning your head or cupping your ear to focus on a certain sound or speaker
- Watching television or listening to the radio at a much louder volume than others

If you suspect that you have hearing loss, consult your doctor.

Hearing Loss
Most hearing loss is due to aging, noise, head injury, or heredity. The most common cause of noise related hearing loss is an excessively loud workplace. Ninety-nine percent of noise related hearing loss can be prevented.

Canadian Association of Speech-Language Pathologists & Audiologists

Hearing Appointments

DATE	DOCTOR	COMMENTS

Approximately 10% of the general population has a hearing problem.

Canadian Association of Speech-Language Pathologist and Audiologists

Hearing Aids

HEARING AIDS	DATE	NOTES AND DETAILS OF PRESCRIPTION

Have your ears examined at least once every year by your doctor, an audiologist or hearing specialist.

Common symptoms associated with hearing impairment are ringing in the ears, a feeling of pressure in the ears and dizziness. See your doctor if you have these symptoms.

Hearing Aid Help

Hearing Insurance Coverage

The best way to use your insurance coverage effectively is to understand the terms of the policy. Take time to read the policy and note the general coverage on this page.

INSURANCE COMPANY	WHAT'S COVERED	PERCENT COVERED	HOW OFTEN	CLAIMS

Appointments & Symptoms

The average appointment time with a doctor is less than 10 minutes. Only about 5 minutes of that is one on one with the doctor.

Appointments

Prior to any appointment write down your questions for your doctor or other health care professional. It is so easy to forget important questions when you are sitting in a doctor's office.

At the appointment or immediately after, write down the answers you received.

	QUESTIONS / ANSWERS / FOLLOW UP
DATE	
NAME OF DOCTOR / HEALTH CARE PROFESSIONAL	

Write Down Your Questions

People who make a list of their questions are likely to ask more questions, feel more in control, and be more satisfied with the visit and the information they receive.

"Take your life in your own hands, and what happens? A terrible thing: no one to blame."

ERICA JONG, AUTHOR

DATE	
NAME OF DOCTOR / HEALTH CARE PROFESSIONAL	
DATE	
NAME OF DOCTOR / HEALTH CARE PROFESSIONAL	
DATE	
NAME OF DOCTOR / HEALTH CARE PROFESSIONAL	

Appointments, continued

It's your right to ask for a copy of your tests and blood work.

	QUESTIONS / ANSWERS / FOLLOW UP
DATE	
NAME OF DOCTOR / HEALTH CARE PROFESSIONAL	
DATE	
NAME OF DOCTOR / HEALTH CARE PROFESSIONAL	

Make sure you understand what your doctor has told you. Repeat the information back to the doctor and then write it down.

DATE	
NAME OF DOCTOR / HEALTH CARE PROFESSIONAL	
DATE	
NAME OF DOCTOR / HEALTH CARE PROFESSIONAL	
DATE	
NAME OF DOCTOR / HEALTH CARE PROFESSIONAL	

Appointments, continued

Don’t hesitate to ask your doctor for treatment options.

	QUESTIONS / ANSWERS / FOLLOW UP
DATE	
NAME OF DOCTOR / HEALTH CARE PROFESSIONAL	
DATE	
NAME OF DOCTOR / HEALTH CARE PROFESSIONAL	

DATE	
NAME OF DOCTOR / HEALTH CARE PROFESSIONAL	
DATE	
NAME OF DOCTOR / HEALTH CARE PROFESSIONAL	
DATE	
NAME OF DOCTOR / HEALTH CARE PROFESSIONAL	

Symptoms & Injuries

List symptoms or injuries such as headaches, muscle soreness, or unusual tiredness. Keeping this list can provide information on recurring problems or symptoms that may help your doctor diagnose a condition over time and help you take a broader look at your own health.

DATE	SYMPTOM / INJURY	TREATMENT

Why memory fails us:

- we tend to think something occurred more recently than it actually did
- we want to remember so badly that we fill in inaccurate details without realizing it
- we tend to forget more when we are in unfamiliar surroundings

Be Specific

For example, instead of "leg pain" say "sharp pain at right knee when climbing stairs.

Women, you may be in Menopause if you notice:

- A change in your menstrual cycle
- Hot flashes
- Headaches
- Trouble sleeping
- Tiredness
- Urinary problems
- Mood swings
- Pain or lack of lubrication with sex

Men, you may be in Andropause (This is also called ADAM or male menopause), if you experience:

- Decreased strength
- Less energy
- Lower sex drive
- Less joy in life
- Erections are less strong
- Feeling sad and/or grumpy

DATE	SYMPTOM / INJURY	TREATMENT

Medicines, Vitamins & Other Treatments

Medicines

If you have medicine prescribed for you it is important to:

- Take it exactly as prescribed. If you have trouble remembering to take it, buy a pill container (available at drugstores) so you can prepare your pills for the week. Another option is to have the pharmacist organize your daily pills into blister packs by the week or month.
- Know why you are taking it, what the possible side effects are and how to take it.
- Call your pharmacist or doctor for instructions if you miss a dose.
- Finish your prescription unless your doctor tells you otherwise.
- Don't mix medicine with alcohol without first asking your pharmacist or doctor.
- Check medicine expiry dates.
- Report any side effects to your pharmacist and doctor.
- Store medicine as directed and in the original container.
- Talk to your pharmacist and doctor about any questions or issues.

! Do NOT quit taking your medicine without first consulting your doctor!

People often quit taking their medicine after reading about possible side effects. However, the side effects listed on medicine handouts are often inaccurate. They are based on what people have complained about while on the drug, but may or may not be related to the drug. If you think you are experiencing SERIOUS side effects go to the emergency department.

! Studies show that people only take their medicines correctly about 50 percent of the time.

! Consuming grapefruit juice (fresh or frozen) can increase, or less commonly decrease, the effects of some drugs. Ask your pharmacist or doctor if this applies to any of your prescriptions.

Medicines

NAME OF MEDICINE	PRESCRIBING DOCTOR	STRENGTH (mg/pill)	PILLS PER DAY	DATE STARTED	DATE STOPPED
SPECIAL INSTRUCTIONS		NOTES: REASON STARTED/STOPPED, SIDE EFFECTS			

NAME OF MEDICINE	PRESCRIBING DOCTOR	STRENGTH (mg/pill)	PILLS PER DAY	DATE STARTED	DATE STOPPED
SPECIAL INSTRUCTIONS		NOTES: REASON STARTED/STOPPED, SIDE EFFECTS			

NAME OF MEDICINE	PRESCRIBING DOCTOR	STRENGTH (mg/pill)	PILLS PER DAY	DATE STARTED	DATE STOPPED
SPECIAL INSTRUCTIONS		NOTES: REASON STARTED/STOPPED, SIDE EFFECTS			

Medicines, continued

NAME OF MEDICINE	PRESCRIBING DOCTOR	STRENGTH (mg/pill)	PILLS PER DAY	DATE STARTED	DATE STOPPED
SPECIAL INSTRUCTIONS			NOTES: REASON STARTED/STOPPED, SIDE EFFECTS		

NAME OF MEDICINE	PRESCRIBING DOCTOR	STRENGTH (mg/pill)	PILLS PER DAY	DATE STARTED	DATE STOPPED
SPECIAL INSTRUCTIONS			NOTES: REASON STARTED/STOPPED, SIDE EFFECTS		

NAME OF MEDICINE	PRESCRIBING DOCTOR	STRENGTH (mg/pill)	PILLS PER DAY	DATE STARTED	DATE STOPPED
SPECIAL INSTRUCTIONS			NOTES: REASON STARTED/STOPPED, SIDE EFFECTS		

A healthy lifestyle can help to minimize the amount of medicine needed to treat many conditions.

If you're thinking about switching to a generic drug or to another brand, ask your doctor or pharmacist. While its usually okay to switch, some switches can cause problems.

"I am always doing that which I cannot do, in order that I may learn how to do it."

PABLO PICASSO

Nearly 30% of all prescriptions used by pharmacies are a generic brand.

Health Canada

NAME OF MEDICINE	PRESCRIBING DOCTOR	STRENGTH (mg/pill)	PILLS PER DAY	DATE STARTED	DATE STOPPED
SPECIAL INSTRUCTIONS			NOTES: REASON STARTED/STOPPED, SIDE EFFECTS		

NAME OF MEDICINE	PRESCRIBING DOCTOR	STRENGTH (mg/pill)	PILLS PER DAY	DATE STARTED	DATE STOPPED
SPECIAL INSTRUCTIONS			NOTES: REASON STARTED/STOPPED, SIDE EFFECTS		

NAME OF MEDICINE	PRESCRIBING DOCTOR	STRENGTH (mg/pill)	PILLS PER DAY	DATE STARTED	DATE STOPPED
SPECIAL INSTRUCTIONS			NOTES: REASON STARTED/STOPPED, SIDE EFFECTS		

"The greatest discovery of our generation is that human beings can alter their lives by altering their attitudes of mind. As you think, so shall you be."

WILLIAM JAMES, PHILOSOPHER & PSYCHOLOGIST

Medicines, continued

NAME OF MEDICINE	PRESCRIBING DOCTOR	STRENGTH (mg/pill)	PILLS PER DAY	DATE STARTED	DATE STOPPED
SPECIAL INSTRUCTIONS			NOTES: REASON STARTED/STOPPED, SIDE EFFECTS		

NAME OF MEDICINE	PRESCRIBING DOCTOR	STRENGTH (mg/pill)	PILLS PER DAY	DATE STARTED	DATE STOPPED
SPECIAL INSTRUCTIONS			NOTES: REASON STARTED/STOPPED, SIDE EFFECTS		

NAME OF MEDICINE	PRESCRIBING DOCTOR	STRENGTH (mg/pill)	PILLS PER DAY	DATE STARTED	DATE STOPPED
SPECIAL INSTRUCTIONS			NOTES: REASON STARTED/STOPPED, SIDE EFFECTS		

Fill all your prescriptions at the same pharmacy so that they have your complete medicine profile.

NAME OF MEDICINE	PRESCRIBING DOCTOR	STRENGTH (mg/pill)	PILLS PER DAY	DATE STARTED	DATE STOPPED
SPECIAL INSTRUCTIONS			NOTES: REASON STARTED/STOPPED, SIDE EFFECTS		

NAME OF MEDICINE	PRESCRIBING DOCTOR	STRENGTH (mg/pill)	PILLS PER DAY	DATE STARTED	DATE STOPPED
SPECIAL INSTRUCTIONS			NOTES: REASON STARTED/STOPPED, SIDE EFFECTS		

NAME OF MEDICINE	PRESCRIBING DOCTOR	STRENGTH (mg/pill)	PILLS PER DAY	DATE STARTED	DATE STOPPED
SPECIAL INSTRUCTIONS			NOTES: REASON STARTED/STOPPED, SIDE EFFECTS		

Medicines, continued

For your convenience, avoid peak hours at the pharmacies – usually lunch time and the end of the business day.

NAME OF MEDICINE	PRESCRIBING DOCTOR	STRENGTH (mg/pill)	PILLS PER DAY	DATE STARTED	DATE STOPPED
SPECIAL INSTRUCTIONS			NOTES: REASON STARTED/STOPPED, SIDE EFFECTS		

NAME OF MEDICINE	PRESCRIBING DOCTOR	STRENGTH (mg/pill)	PILLS PER DAY	DATE STARTED	DATE STOPPED
SPECIAL INSTRUCTIONS			NOTES: REASON STARTED/STOPPED, SIDE EFFECTS		

NAME OF MEDICINE	PRESCRIBING DOCTOR	STRENGTH (mg/pill)	PILLS PER DAY	DATE STARTED	DATE STOPPED
SPECIAL INSTRUCTIONS			NOTES: REASON STARTED/STOPPED, SIDE EFFECTS		

"Everyone thinks of changing the world, but no one thinks of changing himself."

LEO TOLSTOY, AUTHOR

NAME OF MEDICINE	PRESCRIBING DOCTOR	STRENGTH (mg/pill)	PILLS PER DAY	DATE STARTED	DATE STOPPED
SPECIAL INSTRUCTIONS		NOTES: REASON STARTED/STOPPED, SIDE EFFECTS			

NAME OF MEDICINE	PRESCRIBING DOCTOR	STRENGTH (mg/pill)	PILLS PER DAY	DATE STARTED	DATE STOPPED
SPECIAL INSTRUCTIONS		NOTES: REASON STARTED/STOPPED, SIDE EFFECTS			

NAME OF MEDICINE	PRESCRIBING DOCTOR	STRENGTH (mg/pill)	PILLS PER DAY	DATE STARTED	DATE STOPPED
SPECIAL INSTRUCTIONS		NOTES: REASON STARTED/STOPPED, SIDE EFFECTS			

Over-the-Counter Medicines

Over-the-counter medicine is any medicine you buy without a prescription.

NAME OF MEDICINE	REASON TAKEN	DATES

Be sure to check with your pharmacist or doctor about taking over-the-counter medicines

Non-prescription medicines can interact with prescription medicines. For example, non-steroidal anti-inflammatories can raise blood pressure, working against blood pressure pills.

Examples of over-the-counter medicines include pain killers, cold medicine and allergy medicine.

The use of pain medicine increases with age and on any given day 20 to 30 percent of older adults take pain medicine.

NAME OF MEDICINE	REASON TAKEN	DATES

Vitamins, Minerals & Herbs

Learn about possible side effects or cautions of herbal products and nutritional supplements along with the benefits as you would with any prescribed medicine. Carefully consider why you choose to take the product. Report product use to your doctor so he/she can consider whether it interacts with other medicine and conditions you may have.

Caution: There is a lack of evidence for effectiveness and safety of many herbal products and nutritional supplements. In addition, the active ingredients may not have been conclusively identified nor measured. It is also possible that these products may contain contaminants.

<table>
<tr><th>VITAMIN / MINERAL / HERB</th><th>BRAND</th><th>STRENGTH (mg/pill)</th><th>PILLS PER DAY</th><th>DATE STARTED</th><th>DATE STOPPED</th></tr>
<tr><td></td><td></td><td></td><td></td><td></td><td></td></tr>
<tr><td colspan="3">REASON STARTED</td><td colspan="3">REASON STOPPED</td></tr>
</table>

!

Talk to your pharmacist or doctor to ensure your combination of medicines is safe.

Be careful of combinations of vitamins, minerals, and herbs. For example, Gingko and Vitamin E both have blood-thinning properties.

The Canadian Natural Health Products Act came into effect in January 2004. (The act will be instituted over a 6-year period.)

The act aims to establish good manufacturing practices, products & site licensing, research and the use of health claims for natural health products.

VITAMIN / MINERAL / HERB	BRAND	STRENGTH (mg/pill)	PILLS PER DAY	DATE STARTED	DATE STOPPED
REASON STARTED			REASON STOPPED		

VITAMIN / MINERAL / HERB	BRAND	STRENGTH (mg/pill)	PILLS PER DAY	DATE STARTED	DATE STOPPED
REASON STARTED			REASON STOPPED		

VITAMIN / MINERAL / HERB	BRAND	STRENGTH (mg/pill)	PILLS PER DAY	DATE STARTED	DATE STOPPED
REASON STARTED			REASON STOPPED		

Vitamins, Minerals & Herbs, continued

"To be yourself in a world that is constantly trying to make you something else is the greatest accomplishment."

RALPH WALDO EMERSON

VITAMIN / MINERAL / HERB	BRAND	STRENGTH (mg/pill)	PILLS PER DAY	DATE STARTED	DATE STOPPED
REASON STARTED			REASON STOPPED		

VITAMIN / MINERAL / HERB	BRAND	STRENGTH (mg/pill)	PILLS PER DAY	DATE STARTED	DATE STOPPED
REASON STARTED			REASON STOPPED		

VITAMIN / MINERAL / HERB	BRAND	STRENGTH (mg/pill)	PILLS PER DAY	DATE STARTED	DATE STOPPED
REASON STARTED			REASON STOPPED		

Foods are the best source of nutrients, including vitamins and minerals. However you may need to take a supplement to meet your needs at the different stages of life, under particular conditions (i.e., pregnancy or over 50 years of age or if your food choices are limited).

BC Health Files

VITAMIN / MINERAL / HERB	BRAND	STRENGTH (mg/pill)	PILLS PER DAY	DATE STARTED	DATE STOPPED
REASON STARTED			REASON STOPPED		

VITAMIN / MINERAL / HERB	BRAND	STRENGTH (mg/pill)	PILLS PER DAY	DATE STARTED	DATE STOPPED
REASON STARTED			REASON STOPPED		

VITAMIN / MINERAL / HERB	BRAND	STRENGTH (mg/pill)	PILLS PER DAY	DATE STARTED	DATE STOPPED
REASON STARTED			REASON STOPPED		

Vitamins, Minerals & Herbs, continued

VITAMIN / MINERAL / HERB	BRAND	STRENGTH (mg/pill)	PILLS PER DAY	DATE STARTED	DATE STOPPED
REASON STARTED			REASON STOPPED		

VITAMIN / MINERAL / HERB	BRAND	STRENGTH (mg/pill)	PILLS PER DAY	DATE STARTED	DATE STOPPED
REASON STARTED			REASON STOPPED		

VITAMIN / MINERAL / HERB	BRAND	STRENGTH (mg/pill)	PILLS PER DAY	DATE STARTED	DATE STOPPED
REASON STARTED			REASON STOPPED		

VITAMIN / MINERAL / HERB	BRAND	STRENGTH (mg/pill)	PILLS PER DAY	DATE STARTED	DATE STOPPED
REASON STARTED			REASON STOPPED		

VITAMIN / MINERAL / HERB	BRAND	STRENGTH (mg/pill)	PILLS PER DAY	DATE STARTED	DATE STOPPED
REASON STARTED			REASON STOPPED		

VITAMIN / MINERAL / HERB	BRAND	STRENGTH (mg/pill)	PILLS PER DAY	DATE STARTED	DATE STOPPED
REASON STARTED			REASON STOPPED		

Other Treatments (e.g., acupuncture, massage)

Record any treatments such as physiotherapy, acupuncture, or massage, whether your doctor recommended them, or you started them on your own. Gauge how well it worked for you. Include all treatments to make your health record accurate and complete. Let your doctor and other health care professionals know of these treatments.

TREAMENT	REASON I'M HAVING THE TREATMENT	DATES
RESULTS / COMMENTS		

TREAMENT	REASON I'M HAVING THE TREATMENT	DATES
RESULTS / COMMENTS		

People with back pain are willing to try acupuncture, chiropractic adjustment, massage, meditation, and T'ai Chi to relieve their back pain.

"To exist is to change, to change is to mature; to mature is to go on creating oneself endlessly."

HENRI BERGSON,
FRENCH PHILOSOPHER

TREAMENT	REASON I'M HAVING THE TREATMENT	DATES
RESULTS / COMMENTS		

TREAMENT	REASON I'M HAVING THE TREATMENT	DATES
RESULTS / COMMENTS		

TREAMENT	REASON I'M HAVING THE TREATMENT	DATES
RESULTS / COMMENTS		

TREAMENT	REASON I'M HAVING THE TREATMENT	DATES
RESULTS / COMMENTS		

Other Treatments, continued

TREAMENT	REASON I'M HAVING THE TREATMENT	DATES
RESULTS / COMMENTS		

TREAMENT	REASON I'M HAVING THE TREATMENT	DATES
RESULTS / COMMENTS		

TREAMENT	REASON I'M HAVING THE TREATMENT	DATES
RESULTS / COMMENTS		

TREAMENT	REASON I'M HAVING THE TREATMENT	DATES
RESULTS / COMMENTS		

TREAMENT	REASON I'M HAVING THE TREATMENT	DATES
RESULTS / COMMENTS		

TREAMENT	REASON I'M HAVING THE TREATMENT	DATES
RESULTS / COMMENTS		

TREAMENT	REASON I'M HAVING THE TREATMENT	DATES
RESULTS / COMMENTS		

Planning & People

Planning for the Unexpected

Life, Disability and Critical Illness Insurance

TYPE OF INSURANCE	COMPANY NAME	POLICY NUMBER	POLICY DATE	EXPIRY DATE	INSURANCE AGENT	CONTACT NUMBER	1-800 COMPANY NUMBER

The location of my will:

Enduring Power of Attorney and Living Will

A lot of people make a will to take care of matters when they die. However, many of us haven't thought of how we would be taken care of if we were unable to make decisions. Have your lawyer prepare the following two documents to ensure your financial and healthcare matters are taken care of:

Enduring Power of Attorney

- This document gives the person you appoint the legal power to take over your financial affairs should you become mentally incapacitated.
- The name of this document varies from province to province. Other names for it are: *Representative Agreement for Property or Finances, Springing Power of Attorney, Continuing Power of Attorney, and Power of Attorney During Legal Incapacity.*

Advance Health Care Directive (commonly called a Living Will)

- This document outlines your specific instructions for the kind of medical treatment you do or do not want to receive if you are unable to make your wishes known.
- In this document you can also appoint someone to make sure your instructions are followed.
- The name of this document also varies from province to province. Other names for it are: *Representation Agreement for Health Care, Personal Directive, Health Care Directive, Continuing Power of Attorney for Personal Care, and Authorization to Give Medical Consent.*

People

my family and friends

These are the names and contact information of my closest family and friends. In case of an emergency I would like them to be contacted.

NAME	PHONE NUMBER(S)

"The bond that links your true family is not one of blood, but of respect and joy in each other's life."

RICHARD BACH, AUTHOR

Keep the names and numbers of your family, friends and healthcare team up-to-date for easy reference.

"Walking with a friend in the dark is better than walking alone in the light."

HELEN KELLER

"I get by with a little help from my friends."

JOHN LENNON

"When true friends meet in adverse hour,
Tis like a sunbeam in a shower.
A watery way an instant seen,
The darkly closing clouds between."

SIR WALTER SCOTT

NAME	PHONE NUMBER(S)

my healthcare team

List the names and contact information of your doctors, dentist, and other health care professionals. Keep this list up-to-date.

NAME	SPECIALTY	PHONE
ADDRESS		

NAME	SPECIALTY	PHONE
ADDRESS		

NAME	SPECIALTY	PHONE
ADDRESS		

NAME	SPECIALTY	PHONE
ADDRESS		

NAME	SPECIALTY	PHONE
ADDRESS		

NAME	SPECIALTY	PHONE
ADDRESS		

NAME	SPECIALTY	PHONE
ADDRESS		

NAME	SPECIALTY	PHONE
ADDRESS		

NAME	SPECIALTY	PHONE
ADDRESS		

my healthcare team, continued

NAME	SPECIALTY	PHONE
ADDRESS		

NAME	SPECIALTY	PHONE
ADDRESS		

NAME	SPECIALTY	PHONE
ADDRESS		

NAME	SPECIALTY	PHONE
ADDRESS		

"Look to your health; and if you have it, praise God, and value it next to a good conscience; for health is the second blessing that we mortals are capable of; a blessing that money cannot buy."

IZAAK WALTON

NAME	SPECIALTY	PHONE
ADDRESS		

NAME	SPECIALTY	PHONE
ADDRESS		

NAME	SPECIALTY	PHONE
ADDRESS		

NAME	SPECIALTY	PHONE
ADDRESS		

NAME	SPECIALTY	PHONE
ADDRESS		

Notes & Resources

Use this space to jot down your personal thoughts and plans.

"The thing always happens that you really believe in; and the belief in a thing makes it happen."

FRANK LLOYD WRIGHT, ARCHITECT

Notes

"Restlessness and discontent are the first necessities of progress."

THOMAS EDISON

Notes

"Obstacles are those frightful things you see when you take your eyes off the goal."

HANNAH MOORE, PLAYWRIGHT, & PHILANTHROPIST

"Perhaps love is like a resting place, A shelter from the storm, It exists to give you comfort, It is there to keep you warm, And in those times of trouble, When you are most alone, The memory of love will bring you home."

JOHN DENVER

Resources

General

Canadian Health Network: www.canadian-health-network.ca (Health Canada and its affiliates, Canadian professional organizations, provide general health information)

Government of Alberta: Healthy U: www.healthyalberta.com (Current information from Alberta Health and Wellness about healthy choices and factors that affect health)

The Canadian College of Family Physicians: www.cfpc.ca (Patient information on a variety of topics)

Health Canada: www.hc-sc.gc.ca (Government of Canada health information and recommendations)

Health Protection Branch (HPB) of Health Canada: www.hc-sc.gc.ca/hpfb-dgpsa (Canadian federal agency that assures the safety and effectiveness of a range of products)

Heart and Stroke Foundation of Canada: www.heartandstroke.ca (Healthy living tips. Information on heart disease and stroke) (Take the online questionnaire to assess your risk of heart attack and stroke and make an action plan)

Centers for Disease Control and Prevention: www.cdc.gov (United States federal agency with information on many health topics)

U.S. Food and Drug Administration (FDA): www.fda.gov (United States federal agency that assures the safety and effectiveness of a range of products)

UC Berkeley Wellness Letter: www.berkeleywellness.com (From the University of California, Berkeley. It translates leading-edge research into practical advice for daily living. The Wellness Cookbook and Wellness Foods A to Z are available from this site.)

Mayo Clinic: www.mayoclinic.com (Health and illness information. Free weekly newsletters.)

Vitality

Balance

Balance TV: www.balancetv.ca (Morning television show on CTV, hosted by a doctor, various health and wellness topics)

Feeling Good: The New Mood Therapy by David Burns (Problem solving and coping methods for people with depression)

Meditations for Living in Balance by Anne Wilson Schaef (Daily solutions for those who do too much)

Self Nurture by Alice D Domar PhD and Henry Dreher (Learning to Care for Yourself as Effectively as you Care for Everyone Else)

Self Matters by Dr. Phil McGraw (Learn what matters to you and how to live true to yourself)

The Joy of Not Working by Ernie J. Zelinski (A book for the retired, unemployed, and overworked - about finding your life's passions)

The Simple Living Guide by Janet Luhrs (Strategies-Stories-Resources-Inspiration)

Healthy Eating

Dietitians of Canada: www.dietitians.ca (Promotes health through food and nutrition. Analyze your diet with the electronic meal planner. Find a dietitian.)

American Dietetic Association: www.eatright.org (Articles, links and tips on nutrition)

Canadian Food Information Council: www.ccfn.ca (Scientific articles on current food, food safety and nutrition topics)

Canada's Food Guide to Healthy Eating: To receive a free copy of the guide call 1.613.954.5995 or order online at: www.hc-sc.gc.ca/hpfb-dgpsa/onpp-bppn/order_form_e.html

Activity

Canada's Physical Activity Guide to Healthy Active Living: To receive a free copy of the guide call 1.888.334.9769 or order online at: www.paguide.com

Canadian Fitness and Lifestyle Research Institute: www.cflri.ca (Lifestyle Tips columns offer encouragement and practical suggestions for integrating physical activity into daily life.)

Chatelaine Walking Clubs: www.chatelaine.com/health/walkingclubs (Free fitness club for motivation and support)

Sleep

Canadian Sleep Society: www.css.to (Information on sleep disorders and sleep centres in Canada)

National Sleep Foundation: www.sleepfoundation.org (American sleep organization. Take a test to see if you have a sleep disorder)

Healthy Weight

Tufts University Nutrition Navigator: www.navigator.tufts.edu (Provides links and rates nutrition websites)

The Ultimate Weight Solution by Dr. Phil McGraw (Dr Phil's 7 keys to weight loss)

Thin for Life by Anne M. Fletcher (10 weight loss keys from people who have lost and kept it off. Written by a dietitian)

The Prevention Lose Weight Guidebook edited by the Prevention Magazine editors

The Complete Idiot's Guide to Losing Weight by Susan McQuillian, RD and Edward Saltzman, MD (Set clear goals based on realistic approaches to eating. Written by a dietitian and doctor.)

Dieting for Dummies by Jane Kirby and the ADA (Balancing healthy eating and exercise for a lifetime. Written by a dietitian in conjunction with the American Dietetic Association.)

Alcohol, Tobacco, Drugs

Centre for Addiction and Mental Health: www.camh.net (Mental health and addiction information. Press releases on current topics.)

Alcoholics Anonymous: www.alcoholics-anonymous.org (Support group for alcoholics and their families. Resources and contact information.)

Narcotics Anonymous: www.na.org (Support group for narcotics users and their families. Resources and contact information.)

Vitals

High Blood Pressure

The Canadian Hypertension Society: www.hypertension.ca (High blood pressure information for the public and health professionals)

Cholesterol

National Cholesterol Education Program: www.nhlbi.nih.gov/health/public/heart/chol (Information on cholesterol from the National Heart, Lung and Blood Institute of the United States)

Diabetes

Canadian Diabetes Association: www.diabetes.ca (The online resource for people with, and affected by, diabetes and for healthcare professionals treating those affected by the disease)

Osteoporosis

Osteoporosis Society of Canada: www.osteoporosis.ca (Information and support for the prevention and treatment of osteoporosis. Calculate how much calcium you are taking in.).

National Osteoporosis Foundation: www.nof.org (Fighting osteoporosis and promoting bone health in United States)

Cancer

Cancer Society: www.cancer.ca (Cancer information and resources)

National Cancer Institute, U.S. National Institutes of Health: www.cancer.gov (Prevention, diagnosis and treatment of cancer)

Vaccinations

Health Canada, Vaccination Record: www.hc-sc.gc.ca/pphb-dgspsp/publicat/cig-gci/index.html (The Canadian Immunization Guide)

The Canadian Coalition for Immunization Awareness & Promotion: www.immunize.cpha.ca (Provides links to Provincial and Territorial Immunization sites)

Dental, Eye & Hearing

Canadian Dental Association: www.cda-adc.ca (Information, tips and resources on dental health)

The Canadian Association of Optometrists: www.opto.ca (Information, tips and resources on eyesight)

Canadian Association of Speech-Language Pathologists & Audiologists: www.caslpa.ca (Information, tips and resources on hearing and speech)

American Hearing Aid Associates: www.ahaanet.com (Information on hearing loss and hearing aids)

Medication, Vitamins & Other Treatments

Canadian Pharmacists Association: www.pharmacists.ca (Information on medication and treatment of disease and conditions)

US National Institute of Health (NIH): National Center for Complementary and Alternative Medicine: www.nccam.nih.gov (Complementary and Alternative Medicine information, alerts and advisories and resources)

The University of Pittsburgh: The Alternative Medicine Homepage: www.pitt.edu/~cbw/altm.html (Complementary and Alternative Medicine resources maintained by the University of Pittsburgh)

The Desktop Guide to Complimentary and Alternative Medicine. edited by Dr. Edward Ernst, Director of Complementary Medicine, Department of Complementary Medicine, University of Exeter, UK (Provides a review of research evidence on 64 popular forms of complementary and alternative medicine (CAM) and 38 common conditions frequently treated with CAM. Each section is designed to enable quick decision-making.)

Motherisk: www.motherisk.org (Evidence-based information about the safety or risk of drugs, chemicals and disease during pregnancy and lactation.)

Notes

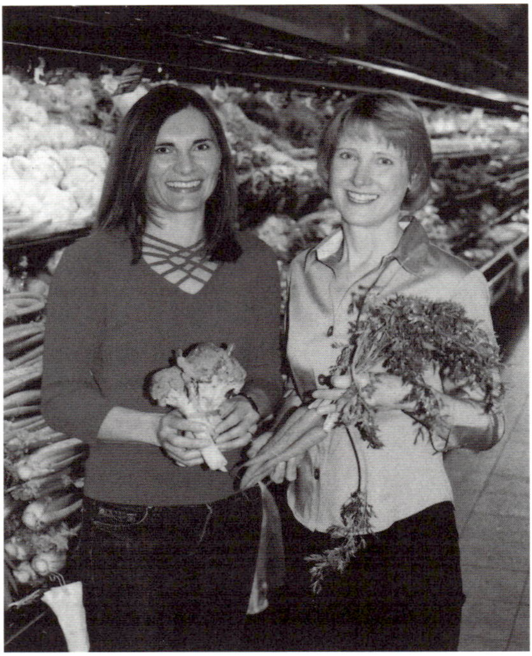

Lorna (left) and Bev (right). Photo taken in the Calgary Co-op Midtown Market by Gerard Sinanan.

About the Authors

Beverly Whitmore, a Registered Dietitian and Lorna Milkovich, a Registered Nurse first collaborated as team members of a leading edge high blood pressure lifestyle treatment clinic in Calgary, Alberta. Through this experience, Bev and Lorna learned what motivates pople to live healthier lives.

Bev has led innovation through project work in redesign of nutrition services, promotion of the health benefits of barley flour and facilitating media relations with health professionals. Lorna specializes in healthcare communication and sidelines as a screenwriter. She has nursed in a variety of settings from intensive care to psychiatry.

Bev and Lorna are co-authors of the Canadian Best Seller *Taking Control of Your Blood Pressure: Steps to a healthier lifestyle.*